HALF-ASSED

a weight-loss memoir

Jennette Fulda

SEAL PRESS

Half-Assed
A Weight-Loss Memoir

Copyright © 2008 Jennette Fulda

Published by
Seal Press
A Member of the Perseus Books Group
1700 Fourth Street
Berkeley, CA 94710

Library of Congress Cataloging-in-Publication Data

Fulda, Jennette.
  Half-assed : a weight-loss memoir / by Jennette Fulda.
    p. cm.
  Includes bibliographical references.
  ISBN-13: 978-1-58005-233-7
  ISBN-10: 1-58005-233-9
  1. Fulda, Jennette. 2. Overweight women—United States—Biography. I. Title.

RC628.F85 2008
362.196'3980092—dc22
[B]
                              2007049499

The events described in this book are true as I remember them, which is as close to the truth as I can ever get. Some names and identifying details have been changed to protect innocent dental hygienists, English teachers, and others.

9 8 7 6 5 4 3

Cover design by Kate Basart
Interior design by Tabitha Lahr
Printed in the U.S.A.
Distributed by Publishers Group West

To Mom, Jim, and Tom.
You guys are the half of myself that
I hope I never lose.

CONTENTS

CHAPTER 1

A History of Fatness

Yellow noodles of fat spilled out of Ms. Ribbit's gut. It wasn't what I was expecting. The textbook featured a precisely drawn diagram of internal organs, clearly defined and colored in neatly between the lines. There wasn't supposed to be any fat. Ms. Ribbit either needed liposuction or someone had stuffed her with Ramen noodles before a shipping error diverted her from the nearest French restaurant to Mrs. Anderson's biology class.

"Ew! That is disgusting!" the boy standing next to me said. Then he started chuckling. The boy's name is forgotten like the names of dozens of boys from my youth, though their words are far more memorable.

"We have the fattest frog ever!" He smacked the table in laughter and pointed out our frog's flayed guts to another nameless boy at the next table. "I guess she took too many trips to the IHOP!"

I looked down at Ms. Ribbit. Metal pins speared her four legs, crucifying her to the dissection tray and displaying her white belly in the most vulnerable of positions. Naked and dead, her guts spilling into the sky, she made it hard to imagine we could devise a way to insult her further, but grade school boys were creative.

I looked down at the flab around my tummy and the thickness of my thighs. I noticed the slight chubbiness of my fingers that held the scalpel. Then I looked back into Ms. Ribbit's glassy, black eyes.

"I'm sorry," I whispered. "I know exactly how you feel."

Then I continued to cut.

I don't remember when I first realized I was fat. I just always was. I do remember the first time someone called me fat. Unsurprisingly, it happened at the beach.

I was about eight years old, a number as round and curvy as I eventually became, when a girl my age and my size stopped me as I was frolicking among the waves in my hot pink bathing suit. She asked me to play, so we started building sand castles using cracked plastic buckets. I got up to retrieve some wet sand near the waterline to add a turret to the east tower. My kneeling playmate pushed herself up against the shifting sand and stumbled behind me.

"Hey, where are you going?" she asked, slightly panicked.

"I just needed to get some more sand," I replied.

"Oh, okay," she said, staring at me for a moment. "We fat girls need to stick together."

Oh my God. Had she just called me fat? I gave her a look up and down. Was I as chubby as she was? Looking back at photos from that trip, I have to admit I resembled a morbidly obese flamingo. Regardless, I couldn't believe she'd actually said that. How could she call me fat? Shouldn't she realize how much that hurt?

"Uh, I gotta go," I said and dashed back to the safety of my parents' beach towel, leaving my fat friend alone and our sand castle sinking into the growing floodplain.

I hadn't been a fat baby. I'd entered this world at eight pounds, five ounces, although I eventually came close to leaving it at 372 pounds.

By fifth grade I was clearly aware of my growing problem. When I was ten, I filled out a questionnaire for school that went like this:

If you could change one thing about your appearance, it would be?
"I would be thinner."

Too bad my answers to the next questions were as follows:

If you could change one thing about your food, it would be?
"I'd have more junk food."

What do you usually do after school?
"Play video games and watch TV."

It'd be nice if I had a good scapegoat for my obesity. I did come from a family of fat people. I could blame their second-rate DNA, except my older brother was thin. He was the errant piece of data screwing up the bell curve of blame. When my mother, father, younger brother, and I were in an elevator, we'd do quick math upon seeing the warning sign, DO NOT EXCEED 2,000 POUNDS. But my older brother was no threat to the system of pulleys and cables. I don't know how he managed it. I should have checked his closet for a secret minifridge stocked with baby carrots and celery.

Sadly, I didn't have a strange disorder to be documented in medical textbooks. I was never sexually abused and driven to build a fat suit of armor for protection. My mother never once nagged me about my weight or put me on a diet, saving me thousands of dollars on therapy. This was great and all, but it left me without any good fall guys. If you're fat, you definitely need a scapegoat or a glandular problem.

The truth is, I was a big, fat cliché. I ate too much and most of my exercise involved walking from the couch to the refrigerator between commercial breaks. I stole the last piece of pie. I went back for a third slice of cake. I ate all the Girl Scout cookies and I probably would have eaten the Girl Scout too if she had been covered in chocolate, caramel, and coconut flakes.

In fourth grade we experimented on a pair of white rats. One rat drank from a bottle of sugar water while the other was given plain H_2O. One of the rats got fat and the other didn't. Obviously I was supposed to learn something about health and nutrition from this lesson, but I just learned that rats like to poop in your hand when you try to weigh them. I never thought about those mice and I never thought about what I ate. When I was hungry I munched on whatever I wanted to, be it half a loaf of Italian bread or a bunch of grapes in the bottom of the crisper drawer.

Every Sunday my parents would buy chocolate-covered, cream-filled éclairs, a reward for attending church without faking rapture to break up the boredom. On my birthday I was sure to get the corner piece of cake, coated in frosting on three sides and topped with a gigantic sugar rose. In my early teens I learned to make fudge off the side of a cocoa powder box and made more batches than the local bakeries. Candy making could be a tricky exercise. Wait too long to pour the bubbling concoction and you'd spend the evening scrubbing hardened sugar crystals out of a pan instead of snuggling up with a square of creamy walnut fudge. I learned exactly when to pour the fudge, just when the surface started to lose its gloss, right when I could no longer see the faint reflection of my double chin in the batter.

That was how we ate at my house. There was rarely anything to contrast against my experience. I got a small inkling of the differences when I visited my friend Justine's house, where they didn't wear shoes on the immaculately clean carpets and they didn't keep soda in their refrigerator. What did they drink? Water? When they offered me a beverage, I had to make do with juice that lacked any carbonated bubbles. When I ate dinner at my friend Cristy's house, I was confused when her mother offered me dark brown bread. I didn't know bread came in colors other than white. The "normalness" of my diet could only be judged by comparing it to someone else's, and I didn't do much comparing. Even if I had noticed that I was eating far too many donuts, realizing the problem doesn't instantly fix it. Diagnosing yourself with a cold doesn't clear your nasal passages.

I didn't sit around all day licking beaters and waiting for my skin to graft to the polyester couch either. I never held my birthday party at McDonald's, nor did I get the Easy-Bake Oven and the snow cone maker I wanted for Christmas. We ate cookies, but we also ate cauliflower. My mom always served a vegetable with every meal, and I got a lot of exercise roller-skating around the basement to Janet Jackson and Paula Abdul songs one summer while I tried not to sail into load-bearing walls. I bonded with my mother by mixing batches of brownie dough in the kitchen but also by riding down to the beach with her in my Big Wheel, sweating and pedaling fast enough to make the fluorescent flag behind me flap wildly in the wind.

Our bathroom featured aquamarine porcelain speckled with paint flakes from the ceiling, but no scale. I discovered how much I weighed only on the occasional trips to the doctor's office. By middle school, that number was 160 pounds.

"Don't worry," the man in the white coat wearing a stethoscope for a necklace told me. "You'll grow into it."

I was unconvinced.

By high school, I found myself exhaling when the nurse slid the heavy iron weight up the white markers on the analog scale, hoping that the rush of air out of my lungs would drop at least an ounce or two off the number. She pushed the lead weight past the 100 mark, then the 150, and finally the dreaded 200 marker. She moved it slowly out of courtesy. It was more polite than slamming it to the far right immediately, which would have saved us time but not embarrassment.

I was one of the fattest people in my class. I'd stopped wearing hot pink bathing suits, fearing bright colors might draw unwanted attention to my size. Instead I spent my senior year of high school wearing baggy, flannel shirts, as though plaid were a form of fat camouflage, the vertical and horizontal lines making onlookers dizzy enough to distract them from my size.

I feared school bus emergency drills. Twice a year we'd have to jump out the back of the bus from three terrifying feet above the ground. Two boys were usually recruited to help students off. When I thought of the terror I would see in their eyes when they had to help me off, my heart rate would rise as if there really were a fire on the bus. What if I stumbled and tackled one of them onto the black pavement? Then we really would need an ambulance.

As I aged, my weight was like the stock market—it had its ups and downs, but on average it trended upward. My first recession came during marching band camp, which drained some fat cells, but unfortunately also drained my patience. I threw up after the first day of practice while waiting at a red light, upchucking rescrambled eggs into a barf bag that my mother had stolen from our last airplane trip (just in case). Later I suffered a spontaneous nosebleed on the field. Then I rubbed a patch of flesh off my heel by wearing ill-fitting marching shoes. Near the end of the season, I had to drag my sorry ass to the shade of the conductor's podium after nearly collapsing from heat stroke.

All this and I still didn't get a PE credit.

I lasted only a year before I turned in my brocade jacket and feathered hat. Thus ended my only youthful flirtation with anything resembling organized exercise. I suspected the band leaders wanted me to leave, though I might have just been suffering from fat girl paranoia: the secret belief that everything that went wrong could be blamed on my fat. I was too breathless to play during the second half of the routine. Several times the camp leaders mentioned that we would drop out of the AAA division and into the less competitive AA division if just one person quit. I held out for the whole season, blood in my shoes be damned.

By the end of high school, I was pushing 260 pounds. I decided the time between high school and college would be a great period to lose weight since few people at my new school would know how fat I'd been. I could adopt a whole new identity and no longer be "the fat girl." I started walking on my dad's treadmill in the basement. I needed to weigh myself, but I didn't have a scale, so I went to the doctor's office every week during my brother's allergy shot to use the one there. I sat between sniffling children and toy trains every Wednesday, managing to lose forty pounds without changing my diet or catching chicken pox.

Too bad no one told me college would be a twenty-four-hour buffet. The dorm's convenience mart was the only store open late at night, stocked with snack cakes, ice cream pints, and chocolate milk. The closest grocery store was about a mile away. It was clearly entrapment. I ran out of money on my meal card before the semester was over, whereas my roommate started buying her friends lunch so she would use all her funds before they expired. I didn't think I was eating more than anybody else, but the negative cash balance on my meal ticket implied otherwise. Was I eating away homesickness or did overweight underclassmen simply need more calories than skinnier students? Ever the overachiever, I gained the freshman fifty.

The university's exercise center was across campus from my dorm room. I reasoned that by the time I got to the center, I would have exercised enough that I'd have to head back to my room. In some twisted form of logic, this convinced me that I shouldn't bother going at all.

I registered for an 8:00 AM advertising class that was booked in an auditorium too small for all the students. Two weeks into classes we were moved to a lecture hall. It was full of tables with mesh wire baskets hanging underneath and swivel seats mounted on poles a fixed distance away from the tables. I turned one of the yellow plastic chairs to the left and sat down, letting out a grunt when the shiny silver wires of the basket pressed into my thighs like string around sausage. I got up and sat on the stairs in the back of the room for the rest of the lecture, avoiding eye contact with the other students. I was prepared to explode in a rant about inadequate seating if anyone accused me of blocking the exits or violating the fire code, assuming I didn't break into tears first. That afternoon I dropped the class. I didn't need to take a stupid advertising course anyway.

I could have learned something from my freshman roommate, Karen, who did abdominal workouts on our floor. This was brave of her. We vacuumed only once a semester, and one afternoon I'd seen a cockroach as big as my thumb scuttle across the floorboards. I didn't think great abs were worth the possibility that a roach might scurry across your face. I was fascinated by her dedicated workout schedule. My family had a committed relationship with the VCR too, but it involved Blockbuster videos, not exercise tapes. Did other people exercise as much as Karen did? We had sent each other introductory letters before the semester started. In mine I made sure to mention that I was fat, as if this were something she needed to be warned about, like leprosy. I watched her do crunches from the bottom bunk. The top bunk had been out of the question for me. I feared I would break the frame and asphyxiate my bunkmate in my sleep.

"I'm thinking of changing my major," she said between leg raises.

"Oh, really?" I asked her. Her foot was getting dangerously close to knocking over the textbook I'd carefully balanced beside the bed to hide my secret stash of Ho Hos hidden underneath. "What to?" Mentally I added, "And move your foot slightly to the left, would you?"

"Foreign language and international economics," she replied as she got up. The instructor on her video kept yelling out commands until she stopped the tape. I couldn't tell if he were German or Austrian or perhaps an alien from a planet with very high gravity, which would explain his muscular physique.

"I've got to see my advisor about it, but I'm going to run first," she said as she grabbed a ponytail holder and put her hair back. I avoided putting my hair back like that because I was afraid it would accentuate my fat face. Big hair made it look smaller. "See ya later," she said as she dashed out the door.

I still didn't have a major. A friend had innocently asked what I wanted to do with my life after college and I'd started hyperventilating on her parents' sofa. At least I was still in school. A girl on the fourth floor who was fatter than me had dropped out after the first week. I wondered if she'd felt out of place because of her size. I reached under the bed for the Ho Hos. Sometimes I'd buy a box of the chocolate cupcakes and eat it alone in two days to dull the stress of my uncertain future. I didn't want anyone else to know about my bingeing because I didn't want to share my emotional problems or my cupcakes with anyone. It was bad enough that the curly-haired clerk at the convenience store had to know. I thought of him as my sugar dealer.

Perhaps if I'd rewound that tape and done some sit-ups myself, I could have averted the stretch mark that I saw on my left inner elbow as

I ripped open the cellophane on my Ho Ho. I'd seen it for two semesters now whenever I rested my head in my hands or laid my arms on a desk. It was a bright pink line that ran for an inch on my otherwise vampire-pale skin. I traced it with my finger during boring lectures. I was tempted to take a red permanent marker to my flesh and add two horizontal strokes, making it a scarlet "F" for fat.

Stretch marks on my belly or breasts were easily hidden with shirts and jeans, and no one ever saw the red, sweaty, chafed mark running beneath my gut flab. My dorm had changing-room stalls that hid my body from sight during showers. I had lots of stretch marks, but only the ones on my breasts were welcome. I may have been a big girl, but I had a small chest. It was impossible to find a bra with a large band size and a small cup size. So I wore bras that didn't fit or struggled with bra-strap extenders that altered the proper alignment of the straps, causing them to constantly slip off my chubby shoulders. I wanted clothes that fit.

Eventually I stopped spending my money on Twinkies at the school's convenience store, but only because I took time off after sophomore year. I couldn't keep filling my schedule with classes like Japanese film or linguistics forever. My new exercise program included surfing the Internet and running through the anime block on the Cartoon Network.

I spent a lot of time walking in place on our treadmill, traveling nowhere. I probably lost weight, but I still didn't own a scale and couldn't measure the loss. I'd bought a scale before college, but it had drowned in a basement flood and I never replaced it. Before its untimely death, I stepped on it only to sadly discover I weighed 270 pounds, which made me mutter, "Why don't I just go for 300?" There was something appealing about hitting a round number, but just as I couldn't commit to a major, I couldn't fully commit to being fat. I was too poor and too scared to buy a new scale because most of them didn't measure over 300 pounds. I didn't want to know if my problem with gravity had become that bad.

The treadmill survived the flood, but it broke during my lost summer. When my father decided it was too expensive to replace, I felt as if I were being sentenced to fatness forever. I could have started walking around the block, but my neighborhood had reckless drivers and no sidewalks. That was my excuse, but in reality I was too ashamed of my size to exercise in public. I could stand the chafing as my thighs rubbed together, but the piteous glares of neighbors would have rubbed me the wrong way.

Thus ended another period of yo-yo exercising. Strangely, I never yo-yo dieted. I never went on a diet at all, which was either completely boneheaded of me or completely brilliant, depending on how you look at it. I had heard that yo-yo dieting could mess with your metabolism, causing you to gain back even more weight and making it harder to lose weight in the future.[1] Recent studies have shown that this may not be true, although weight cycling might weaken your immune system.[2] Regardless, staying away from diet shakes and rice cakes saved me the emotional exhaustion that comes from trying dozens of fad diets and failing them all. I should have made an effort to eat a more balanced diet, though. I was under no delusions that the bag of peanut butter cups in my desk drawer was part of a healthy eating program, despite studies showing that chocolate can lower blood pressure.[3]

Even though I wanted to eat better, I was suspicious of people trying to sell me a book or a plan. They obviously had something to gain if I bought it. I was cheap and didn't want to pay for an institutionalized program like Weight Watchers. If anyone was going to get paid for losing weight, it should be me. I'd be doing all the work. Those programs never released statistics on how many people were able to lose weight and keep it off, which made me wonder if they worked at all. I'd heard dieting usually included food deprivation, which I wasn't willing to try. It also seemed really complicated. I didn't think I could count calories or keep track of the carbohydrate/fat/protein ratios for all of my meals, nor did I want to.

The people who wrote diet books couldn't agree on anything anyway, so I was hesitant to trust them. Some authors said carbs were bad; others said they were good. For several years everyone thought fat would make you fat, but then they decided maybe that wasn't true.[4] Diets were like religions. There were hundreds of them and everyone thought his or hers was the right one. Ultimately it was just a matter of faith. I wanted something solid. I wasn't interested in dieting.

I didn't want to fail either. I was already fat, but if I tried a diet and it didn't work I'd be a big fat loser too. It was safer not to commit to a plan. Even when I started exercising the summer before college, I never made a formal announcement about it. My family knew what I was doing when they heard the treadmill in the basement and saw me tag along on boring doctor visits, but if I could have exercised and weighed myself in secret I would have. If no one knew I had tried, it would be far less embarrassing when I failed.

After two semesters off, I started college again and eventually found a part-time desk job designing print materials. I got to create business cards while sitting on my butt all day, saving my feet from the pain of standing for hours on end, as the cashiers did. I moved into an apartment, and I walked around the complex regularly, though only during the day. I was hesitant to venture into the neighborhood at night, which stopped me from making late-night junk food runs. I decided I'd rather have a dead craving for a jar of frosting than be dead. A month of snowfall stopped me from walking and I continued to get fatter. At least the extra insulation kept me warm.

I had always hoped I would someday become thin, just as I'd idly hoped I would someday become a rock star. But my pants were still as big as a potato sack and I wasn't singing rock anthems to screaming groupies. Was this thin thing ever going to happen for me? I was in my twenties and I felt like time was running out to enjoy being thin if I ever lost the weight. I toyed with the idea that I might have deep-seated emotional issues that were leading me to overeat, but my internal searching didn't turn up much. I hated the fat, but I didn't hate myself. I thought I was a rather intelligent, witty person if you got to know me. There was just a lot of me to know. The fat was like a separate entity, not a true part of me. Those extra fat cells were uninvited guests on my body, just like the infestation of pharaoh ants in my ghetto apartment.

I was pretty shy though, always hiding behind a huge mess of frizzy hair. Fat girls were invisible. Maybe I was making myself fat so I could hide in plain sight? When I tried to figure out why I was so overweight, everything I came up with sounded like an episode of *Dr. Phil* that I would promptly turn off. Sometimes emotional hypotheses seemed like bullshit explanations. They were simple answers to complex problems. I just needed to walk more and make sure I wasn't walking past an ice cream truck. But if it were that simple, how come I hadn't been able to do it yet? What was I waiting for?

During my senior year of college, my father drove off for the coast, stopping only to mail a letter that did little to explain why he was divorcing my mother. I guess I wasn't the only one doing some soul searching. In German, the word *kummerspeck* is used to describe the weight you gain from emotional overeating. It literally translates to "grief bacon." If I weren't staring at my powered-down computer in the dark wondering what had gone wrong in my parents' seemingly perfect marriage, I was probably munching on the orange-chocolate sandwich cookies I'd recently discovered in the candy aisle. No revelations were printed on the shortbread.

If he'd left when I was eleven instead of twenty-one, I could blame my obesity on him. But I was already pushing 350 pounds by the time he took off, so I can assign only twenty pounds of weight to his eventual exit. I could try to divvy up the blame for the rest of the excess weight too—thirty pounds for sodas, forty for a slow metabolism, and at least five for finals week. That leaves thirty pounds for unresolved emotional issues, fifty-five for ignoring nutritional information, twenty for an urban infrastructure that didn't require me to walk anywhere, and ten wild card pounds left over to blame on everything else. Assigning blame wasn't going to make me thin or change what my dad had done.

At my college graduation, I was chosen to carry the departmental banner into the ceremony. Otherwise I would have skipped the whole ordeal. I was given the largest size robe, but it was still tight around my waist. While many of my fat photos stimulate the pain center of my brain, looking at my graduation photos makes electroshock therapy seem like a spa treatment. No one looks thin wearing a black sheet, especially not the 372-pound girl.

At the smaller departmental ceremony later on, I had to stand up to be recognized for an honor. I felt enormous.

That's because I was.

CHAPTER 2

Living Large

One of the prerequisites for being a fat girl, besides owning at least one pair of pants with an elastic waistband, is that you must have horrible fat stories. If someone has not made you feel small for being so big, you won't be allowed into the fat-girl clubhouse, even if you can't fit through the door frame anyway. I sometimes feel as if I didn't live up to my full discrimination potential because I don't have as many fat-girl horror stories as some women. I really should have left my room more often.

The earliest fat shaming I can recall occurred in middle school, a time in my life I have worked hard *not* to recall. I prefer to believe that the universe skipped past that time like the lame track on an otherwise stellar CD. In middle school, the student body was corralled like cattle onto the bleachers in the gym until the bell rang ten minutes before classes started. In between weekly brawls, fat girls made for good entertainment.

One morning a boy sidled up to me and tapped me on the shoulder, getting dirty boy germs on my shirt. "Hey, see my friend over there?" he asked, as if to verify I was not blind as well as fat. I turned and looked at a pack of three boys wearing jeans and shit-eating grins. They were flanked by another guy who held his head in his hands and looked as uncomfortable as I felt. "He really likes you," my attacker said.

I thought so little of my physical attractiveness that I doubt I would have realized if someone actually did hit on me. However, I could tell I was just the big butt of their joke. I turned back to stare at the fascinating air molecules swirling in front of me, wishing I were as invisible as the oxygen I was inhaling in frustrated breaths. The boy continued to stare at me, waiting for some sort of reaction. I wouldn't look at him. He didn't exist. I didn't exist. This wasn't happening. Someday I would become thin and beautiful and I would wreak vengeance on all of these boys, even if I didn't know their names.

Bored with his prey, the boy bounded back up the bleachers. If I could rewrite the story, I would throw in a scene in which I tripped him and then kicked him in the balls.

I was shy, so I didn't venture outside of school much. Most of my time was spent indoors watching other people's lives on television rather than living my own. The brick and drywall of our house became a safe zone from the war fought at school. My brothers never made fun of my fat and my parents never nagged me about it.

Outside of the home, insults could happen anytime, anywhere, at the most unexpected moments, like a roadside bomb exploding. KABOOM! I would suddenly be reminded that I was fat and that I should hang my head in shame toward my potbelly. Insults don't bounce off a jiggly belly as well as the laws of physics and elasticity would have you believe. I'd never talked to the girl across the street who was a year ahead of me at a different high school. Our first verbal exchange didn't make me regret that. As I walked across the driveway to my parents' car, I saw her perched in an open window on the second floor with a friend.

"Jelly roll!" one of them yelled.

I stopped in confusion. "What?" I asked, throwing my question across the street.

"Jelly roll!" they now replied in unison as they started giggling. The words stung as if they'd tossed sticks and stones. Why was she doing this? Weren't there ants that she could burn with a magnifying glass instead? "Jelly roll" wasn't even a good insult. The boys on the bleachers were far more creative.

The next year they moved out after a kitchen fire. I liked to imagine it happened when she was baking jelly rolls.

Sometimes attacks seemed accidental. As I was walking across the school courtyard thinking about my math homework, one of two boys behind me murmured, "Doesn't Jennette have the biggest ass you've ever seen?" Their snickering hit me like shrapnel. The boys on the bleachers wanted to confirm I wasn't blind, and the boys behind me seemed to think I was deaf. Did everyone think fat people were disabled? I *did* have a huge ass, so in a twisted way I was just hearing the facts. But high school boys have a way of wielding the truth as a weapon.

And I never fought back.

Among your fat-girl stories, there is a mandatory requirement of at least one traumatic shopping experience. If you have never been reduced to tears in a dressing room, please check your waist measurement; you may not actually be fat. Or you're one of the handful of fat girls who never had body issues and always rocked your fatness. If so, congratulations; you are way more awesome than the rest of us who let our thunder thighs steal our thunder.

My worst fat-girl shopping experience came near the end of high school, a time when senioritis should have kept me from caring about anything. At graduation the boys and girls wore robes in our school colors, red and white. They arranged our seating so we spelled out the first initial of my school's name. Snap, click, a picture was taken for the guidance counselor's wall to celebrate that he was finally rid of us. The white gowns weren't a solid white, just a cheap, sheer nylon, so the girls had to wear white or pastel dresses under their robes. Comply or risk not participating in the ceremony.

My high school made a 250-pound teenage girl buy a white dress. I should have sued it for child abuse.

I may as well have been searching for a six-toed, purple, hairless yeti since they are far more common than a flattering white dress on a fat girl. After my first unfruitful day of shopping, I wanted to cry all the way home like the little piggy I felt like. Instead, my mother and I rode home in silence. I rolled down the window so the glass wouldn't reflect the image of my fat face. The car pulled into the driveway and I got out as quickly as I could, heading straight for the stairs and my bedroom. I didn't bother turning the lights on. The three hundred-thread-count pillowcase muffled my sobs and absorbed my tears. Shame and self-loathing are best savored in private.

But I still didn't have a dress. The next day my mother and I descended upon the last fat-girl clothing store in the area. If we failed to find something, I was going to march to the department store next door and buy a white bed sheet to wear as a toga.

I shoved metal hangers across metal racks to make nerve-racking screeching sounds. It provided the perfect background sound to accompany the horror I experienced when I turned around. It couldn't be. No. Not now. Not here.

It was my freshman English teacher, Mrs. Warren, with the long black hair that descended her short, squat frame past her butt.

"Jennette, fancy seeing you here!" she bubbled. ·

I stood paralyzed, as if caught in the glare of her shiny, silver, square earrings. I hated seeing teachers outside of school walking around pretending they were normal people with actual lives. Once I had spotted my math teacher at the grocery store and ducked behind a row of diet pills to avoid her. It was the best use for Fen-phen I'd ever found.

"Uh ..." I mumbled. Then my mother swooped to my rescue.

"Hi! I'm Jennette's mom. We met at open house night," she said as she offered her hand to Mrs. Warren. "We're just here shopping for a graduation dress," she continued, as her personality filled the room and I blended into the background.

As they kept gabbing, I started wandering to the dressing rooms with two dresses that might not make me look like the Stay Puft Marshmallow Man's chubby little sister. As I turned the corner, I nearly dropped the clothes hangers in shock.

There, exiting the dressing rooms, was Mrs. Fielding, my current senior English teacher, who taught from her chair because standing all day hurt her feet. I was shopping at the same store as not one, but two, of my English teachers. If they had been math teachers instead, they'd have known the odds against this happening. Mrs. Fielding stepped back in surprise as we locked eyes.

"Jennette, fancy seeing you here!" she said. Then she noticed my entourage and greetings were exchanged. All of us. Together. At the fat-girl store. At the exact same time.

There must have been one killer sale going on.

"Why don't you go and try on those dresses?" my mother said.

"Yeah, we can have a little fashion show and tell you what we think," seconded Mrs. Warren.

At this point my memory goes blank. I can't recall the ordeal of trying on several white dresses for half of the English faculty at Everett

High School. I've read that the mind blocks out traumatic memories for its own protection. I figure it's for the best.

I did finally find a dress that wasn't completely atrocious. I sold it online after eBay was invented. I've never run into my former English teachers while shopping again either, but only because I moved to another state.

Near the end of high school I became friends with Felicity. I liked that she got free movie rentals. She liked that I was fatter than she was.

One easy way to make yourself feel thin is to hang out with someone who is fatter than you. I didn't do this much because not many people could make me feel thin. When I was still only moderately fat in middle school, a girl who was fatter than me moved into a rental house down the street. I can't remember her name. I *can* remember sitting at our out-of-tune piano when what's-her-name appeared next to me. For the first time in my life, I felt small, like a cotton T-shirt that had shrunk three sizes in the dryer. If I'd known how to, I would have played a dramatic minor seventh chord to accompany my shock. Did people feel this tiny when they stood next to me?

I never became good friends with the nameless girl from down the street, but Felicity started calling me a lot our senior year. She was one of only two people who asked me to do stuff in high school to coax me out of my room.

Felicity was pushy and I was a pushover, and so our dysfunctional friendship began. I didn't think she was fat, but like many teenage girls she thought she really needed to lose fifteen pounds. Superman may have x-ray vision, but Felicity could spot a six-ounce weight loss or gain on anyone's body. She would frequently mention who she thought had lost weight. I found this fascinating and disturbing. I wanted to be thinner, but I wasn't betting on the prom queen's dress size. Felicity even joined Weight Watchers for a while. I'm sure all the truly fat girls at her meetings must have wondered what a thin girl like Felicity was doing in their cult.

Felicity and I eventually "broke up" during our first year of college. She was high maintenance and I had gotten to a point where I was afraid to answer the phone. My family was too cheap to get caller ID. I had started avoiding her when I went home for visits and would tell people not to mention that I'd been in town. I was hoping our friendship could just fade out like many high school relationships. I hated conflict and didn't know how to dump her gracefully.

It was also hard because Felicity and I had good times. We weren't friends just because I was fatter than her. She was brave when I was cowardly, passionate when I was hesitant. She was living out loud while I had the volume turned down so I wouldn't disturb my neighbors. She's still the only person I've sung "Girls Just Want to Have Fun" with badly and boldly while driving along the interstate with the windows down.

I eventually sent Felicity an email telling her I thought our friendship had run its course. This still ranks in the top ten shittiest things I have ever done in my life. She at least deserved a phone call, but I knew I'd just break down and start crying over the conflict. In Felicity's life story, I don't doubt that I am credited as "Mean Girl #3."

I fear a high school reunion because Felicity's the kind of person who would slap me. And then throw a drink in my face. And then stab me with a toothpick. We'd sometimes go for walks on the perfectly trimmed grass of the park near my house and talk about how thin we'd be by our high school reunion. I wonder how she'd feel about the fact that I actually did it. She might have done it too. I wonder if it made her feel less miserable about her body, or if after all that walking she ultimately ended up in the same place she started?

Being fat was traumatic, but the food was *amazing*.

I ate like most people would dare to only if an asteroid were scheduled to demolish the planet tomorrow afternoon. I've never been on the set of an XXX video, but I've seen food porn up close and personal. Culinary voyeurism, just like shocking tales of sexual exploits, will make you sit back in stunned silence thinking, "She put a *what* in her mouth?" I didn't get fat because I had mad broccoli cravings. I ate frozen orange juice concentrate straight out of the can. I sucked on spoonfuls of Tang crystals. At restaurants I would grab packets of jellies and jams from the center of the table, peel back the silver covers, and lick the gooey insides off my fingers.

My daily lunch during sophomore year of high school was a box of Everlasting Gobstoppers I bought from the librarians as soon as the bell rang. My breakfast was four slices of whole-wheat bread.

I slathered slices of white bread with butter and ate them raw. If I had thought to sprinkle sugar on top, I would have tried that too. I bought bags of mini-marshmallows and popped the cylindrical puffs into my mouth one by one, counting how many I could dissolve into a gigantic, high-fructose blob without suffocating.

When my family was away for a week, I made a no-bake Oreo cake so I could eat it all myself. I snacked on rocks of brown sugar. I drank maple syrup straight out of the jar until the sugar burned the back of my throat.

And it was *good*.

As freaky as these tawdry excerpts from my childhood food diary are, I didn't eat like this all the time. Incidents involving a collectible Care Bears glass from McDonald's containing equal parts of chocolate syrup and milk are memorable *because* they didn't happen every day. You don't get to be five feet and nine inches tall without having some nutrients in your diet.

I'm not sure why I did these things. I could say it was a way of burying my feelings. I could say it just tasted good and I didn't know better. I could spin some story about how food never judged me. But I don't know if any of those things are actually true. I just know that I ate the whole pizza.

I obviously knew making chocolate frosting as an afternoon snack was wrong; otherwise I wouldn't have secretly made it in the basement with a hand mixer. It was wrong in the same way that downloading MP3s off the Internet is wrong—I could do it without much guilt. If you could eat half a bowl of cookie dough without feeling guilty about the chocolate chips melting in your mouth, wouldn't you? And if we lived in a magical fairyland where cookie dough had zero calories, would there be any reason not to?

After college, I lived with my mom for several years while I paid off credit card debt and college loans. Occasionally she invited people over, people with functioning visual cortexes, people who would see how fat I had become. This wouldn't do.

My relatives were coming over. I obviously needed to hide.

I'd never been social. Even before I'd become fat I'd been the last girl in first grade handing out valentines to all my peers because I didn't know their names. For several years in middle school I refused to answer the phone, which couldn't have had much to do with my fat because my voice didn't sound particularly chubby. In college I wondered if I might have social anxiety disorder, but my research revealed those people were terrified to simply go to the grocery store. Obviously I didn't have that problem.

Once past the 300-pound mark, I avoided seeing old friends and relatives so they wouldn't know how out of control my problem had become. I now lived in a different city and state than where I had gone to high school, so I never ran into old friends at the mall, not that I ever went to the mall. I had outgrown the largest pants at Lane Bryant, so there was no reason to face the packs of skinny teenagers in low-rise jeans. Meeting strangers wasn't any better because I knew the first thing they'd see was my fat, which I found to be rather disgusting. I would look at myself naked in the mirror before I took a shower and try to wash away the self-loathing with the "hard rain" setting on the showerhead. If I felt that way about myself, how could I expect other people not to?

Several of my aunts and uncles were dropping by on their way home from my cousin's Little League game in Bloomington. I wanted to leave the house and hide in the dark of a movie theater, if my butt would fit in the seats. But I stayed and greeted my aunts and uncles at the door for my mother's sake so I wouldn't appear rude. Then I hid in the back den at the first possible moment.

Fifteen minutes went by. Then thirty.

How long were they going to be here? Weren't they in a hurry to get where they were going? I heard my young cousins dashing around the sofa in the living room and decided I need to make a dash for it too. Now. I crept out the back hallway into the garage and into my car. I pushed the button on the automatic garage door opener and left without telling anyone where I was going.

Where *was* I going? How far would I have to drive before I escaped myself? I wasn't so different from my dad after all.

After an hour browsing the dollar bin at Target, I struggled across the parking lot and headed home. I slowed down at the stop sign three lawns from our house. I turned my head left and peered down the street. My mother was talking to my aunt, who was smoking a cigarette, in the front yard. They caught a glimpse of my maroon car and started waving at me.

I took my foot off the brake and kept driving. I'd been made, but I couldn't go back there. They'd invaded my safe zone, my land of denial, the place I felt comfortable being fat. But I had nowhere else to go. I drove and drove. I think I stopped at a Starbucks. Time passed. I drove by our front yard again, and finally all their cars were gone.

I entered our house through the garage so the neighbors wouldn't see me.

"Are you okay?" my mom asked.

"Yeah," I said

"Where did you go? Didn't you see us waving at you?" she asked. "We were worried."

"I'm sorry." I said. "I just had to get away." Too bad it never worked.

What I regret most is all the stories I don't have to tell. I wanted to take a swing dancing class in college, but I didn't go because I couldn't foresee anyone flinging my fat ass into the air. At a birthday party held at a hotel, I lied and said I'd forgotten my bathing suit, which was actually hidden under my Rainbow Brite pajamas in my suitcase. Let's not even talk about the times I tried to play on the teeter-totter.

I was an accomplice in a hate crime against myself. I was a mime feeling up walls that didn't exist but that I thought separated me from the world. I don't have any stories about the high school prom because I didn't go. I could have gone with a gay guy, but I said no, escaping at least one fat-girl cliché. I didn't want to face a ballroom filled with my peers. I didn't think I would look good in a dress either, if I could manage to find one that didn't make me look like a cupcake. I don't particularly regret not going, but I regret that I thought I couldn't go. Even if I were the ugliest, fattest girl on the planet, I didn't owe it to anyone to be pretty and thin.

A decade later, I lost more than a hundred pounds to weigh what I had senior year. I bought a black and pink dress with a delicately embroidered rose on the bodice to wear to a cousin's wedding. It was the fanciest dress I'd ever bought. I was still fat, but I felt stunning. I also looked like a bridesmaid because no one told me the wedding colors were pink and black.

I went through old photos recently trying to figure out how fat I had been at different times in my life. I found one from middle school, back when I felt like a human dump truck. I looked so thin. I wanted to invent a time machine for the sole purpose of going back to smack some sense into myself. You are almost never as fat as you think you are. If I could teach the fat girls of the world one thing, that would be it.

But eventually I got fatter than I'd ever been, and a positive attitude could help me only so much. Some problems had nothing to do with my self-image or what magazine editors in New York put on their covers. When I was morbidly obese, restaurant booths were too small and seat belts didn't always buckle. It was the inverse of the days when I was a child, when kitchen counters were too high and chairs were too big. The world was not sized to fit me. I felt like I didn't belong.

Ironically, while the items in the world frequently seemed too small, the world itself was often too large. One summer I attended a lawn concert on the river and had to walk half a mile to and from the parking lot. I was mortified as people constantly passed me, effortlessly walking by on an evening stroll, while I struggled all 2,600 feet just to reach my car. Out of breath and sweating, I told myself, as I told myself every day of my life, "I really need to lose weight."

That thought was as much a part of my mental routine as thinking *I'm tired* or *I need to clean the litter box.* No matter how good your life is, I suspect everyone has an inner voice that whispers that life isn't quite good enough. It tends to do a lot of talking after high school reunions and unexpected meetings with happily married ex-boyfriends. Mine spent a decade telling me I was a fat ass. It was like watching the TV movie of my life but constantly being interrupted for ads selling self-loathing cream. There was a lot of good programming on my personal television network too, but it doesn't appear in this book. It has been edited for content and to run in the allotted time. I just wanted to recast the lead character as someone thinner.

When I think about how I let myself get so absurdly fat, I think of a box of clothing patterns my mother gave me when I told her I was launching a search and rescue mission for the lost art of sewing. I didn't dive into the box of patterns within the first week I had them, so the box eventually became a part of my apartment's landscape, marking its borders with deep impressions in the carpet. After a week it felt less urgent to pop the lid than it had during the first few days when it was a new thing. Similarly, if I didn't start reading a new book within the first week, it stopped being a book and became a multipaged dust collector for my bookshelf.

When people asked me how I could possibly let myself go, that's how. All that weight was a box of dress patterns in the corner or that library book I renewed for the fourth time. I said I would get to them, but I never did. It became part of my terrain. After a point, so much weight piled up that the task seemed insurmountable. It was the difference between reading one book and reading the entire Library of Congress.

The fat lost its shock value. It didn't scare me like it scares a skinny girl who's just put on ten pounds and can't fit into her favorite jeans. Ten pounds was a trivially small percentage of my overage. Who would notice if I lost only ten pounds? The necessity of losing weight today was no more urgent than it had been yesterday or would be tomorrow. I built up a tolerance. Being fat became normal. It became as much a part of my identity as being the smart one or the girl who was good with computers. Other people were skinny.

Yet the dream of thin never went away. Because it wasn't just the dream to be thin, it was the dream to be happy, to be loved, and to be safe. It was the assurance that life would be okay, that I would be accepted. It meant the power of beauty, over men and other women. This was what being thin meant. It didn't matter if it was true.

At night I would stare at the ceiling wondering how many years my weight was taking off my mattress's lifetime and hoping someday I'd be able to start a sentence with the phrase, "After I lost all that weight after college . . . "

CHAPTER 3

The Snooze Button

It was three o'clock in the morning and I wanted to die.

I was home from college for the weekend and enjoying the familiarity of sleeping in my old bed instead of sharing a bunk in the freshman dorm. That was, until I was awoken by the worst pain I'd experienced in my seventeen years and eleven months on the planet. It felt like heartburn at first, but it quickly intensified to heart-inferno and then became a heart-supernova, threatening to implode in a starburst of pain in my stomach. I began plotting to cut open my chest with my retainer. My orthodontist had left a couple of sharp plastic edges around the rim that could make a clean incision.

Instead I crept to my parents' room and knocked on the door. My mother rushed me to the downtown hospital where I was triaged and asked if I were on drugs or pregnant. When the hospital staff realized I was not yet eighteen, I was sent to the kiddie hospital next door without even receiving a lollipop.

I was wheeled to the adjoining hospital so slowly that my mother was able to move the car and start a conversation with the on-call nurse in the lobby before I arrived. Without the aid of a remote control, I rewound the last ten minutes of my life for repeat viewing: triage, medical questions, and the query as to whether I was a crackhead or knocked up, or better yet, a crackhead with a little crack baby in my womb. People always wanted easy answers.

I waited in the lobby, keeled over in pain, confused why no one seemed to be interested in helping me or at least considerate enough to knock me unconscious with an IV stand. Eventually I was shown to an examining room and asked to lay down on a bed covered in white paper that crinkled and folded awkwardly beneath me. Was I intoxicated? Was there a living being inside of me? The intern asked me those questions as she struggled to feel my organs underneath my layers of fat. She succeeded only in tickling me.

"If a syringe full of heroin and a hard cock will make this pain go away, bring it on," I said. (Actually, I didn't, but I really wish I had.)

It was at this point that I started to question the perfection of the medical system. Doctors are just human, after all, and as fallible as the rest of us. I hoped they were right most of the time, particularly when they were working on me, but the repeated questioning made me wonder if they had any idea what they were doing. My mother inquired twice, "Could it be her gallbladder?" The intern just shook her head no. Our family had a history of gallbladder disease, but I was rather young for it. When the pain finally went away, no thanks to anyone in a white coat, I was told it was probably gas and to take some antacids with simethicone next time.

In the following years I had several attacks similar to that first one but without the chaser of a hospital bill. A couple of weeks before my twenty-third birthday I awoke in the middle of the night to a familiar pain under the right side of my ribs. My internal organs didn't even have the decency to malfunction during normal business hours. I rolled around in bed and moaned for five hours until the doctor's office opened. My general practitioner was cheaper than the ER. When I finally arrived at the office, it took all of a minute for my doctor to determine I was probably having a gallbladder attack. Hardened stones of cholesterol had formed in my gallbladder and were trying to squeeze their way through my common bile duct. It was like trying to shove a cantaloupe through a garden hose.

The doctor prescribed painkillers that made me feel so happy they should have had smiley faces printed on them. I had never done drugs before, but I started to question my elementary school enrollment in Nancy Reagan's "Just Say No" program when the small white tablets quickly killed the nine hours of intense, stabbing agony. While I was glad I no longer wanted to reach into my belly to start ripping out organs, the pain had been an amazingly transcendent experience. I no longer feared childbirth. Pushing a baby out of my vagina sounded like a party with Jell-O shots and cheesecake after this.

Before this attack, my main motivation to be thin was to be drop dead sexy and wear a pair of calf-high leather boots that actually fit around my calves. But as I entered my twenties—or the three hundreds, depending on what I was measuring—I realized the sexiest thing was not being dead.

I had passed the one stone that caused me so much pain, but if there were others, they could become lodged in my bile duct at any time. Several days after my latest attack I went to have an ultrasound on my abdomen to confirm that my problem was indeed gallstones. If so, I would have to schedule surgery to have my gallbladder removed.

I got lost in the hospital's shiny corridors until I finally wandered into the proper waiting room. I squished myself between the arms of a chair, my fat spilling over like a muffin top. I was soon called into a darkly lit room where a technician squirted gel on my stomach and ran a wand over my upper right quadrant. She barely said a word. I never liked small talk, but for the first time in my life I missed the static of empty words.

"Have you eaten today?" she finally asked, staring at the screen with a wrinkled brow.

"No," I replied. She grunted and finished the scan without another word. This couldn't be good. A couple of days later I got the call. I'd have to have my gallbladder removed. It was a pointless body part anyway, like the tonsils and appendix. I went to all the trouble of supplying it with blood and oxygen and all it did was cause me pain. The gall, indeed.

I'm lucky my gallbladder didn't burst and become infected before my diagnosis. Then the doctors would have had to slice me up the side like a sea bass to repair the damage. Instead my surgery would be done laparoscopically, a tiny camera snaked up my abdomen. The surgeons would make four tiny incisions, inflate my belly like an air mattress, and cut the pouch of stones out, sucking them up with a vacuum. They would even give me pictures of the procedure, though the photos looked as if they could have been faked with a pound of boneless chicken breasts and a scalpel.

My mother drove me to the consultation with the surgeon. I sat in the white office with my feet dangling off the end of the firmly padded table, feeling like a child dipping her toe into a potentially deadly ocean. The doctor came in, tall, dark, and friendly, and went over the procedure, accidentally tickling my belly as he showed me where he'd make the incisions. Then he mentioned the elephant in the room. It wasn't Dumbo.

"I know this is probably a sensitive topic, but as your doctor I have to tell you that your current weight is cutting off at least seven years of your life. This puts you at extra risk during surgery." He looked down at his clipboard and back up directly into my eyes. "If you're interested, we've got an excellent weight-loss center with nutritionists and dieticians that can help you lose weight. You might also want to consider weight-loss surgery."

Uh-oh. He'd noticed I was fat. Wasn't it just like a scientist to be observant? At least he was polite, never condescending or judgmental, a hard tightrope for a doctor to walk when confronting a patient about a weight problem. I knew some fat women who avoided going to the doctor because they didn't want to be lectured about their weight, as if it were something they could fix as easily as dinner. His good manner could almost make me forget that he probably had incentive to recommend me to the in-house surgical center.

I could feel my cheeks and chest heat up, reddening as they always did when I was anxious or embarrassed. Yet I was oddly relieved. Someone had noticed my problem. We didn't really talk about fat in my house. The closest I'd gotten to having a conversation about obesity with my mother was when I'd snuggled against her cushy body during a long car trip as a kid and told her she made a good pillow. This was before the phrase "obesity epidemic" was in every other health news story. Almost everyone in my family had a weight problem and none of us wanted to talk about it, because none of us knew how to fix it. I certainly never wanted to approach my parents and ask them, "Hey, why'd you guys let me get so fat?" We weren't oblivious to the issue. My mother joined Weight Watchers once, though I didn't know it at the time, but the points system couldn't fix this problem point in my family.

Almost no one outside of the family was bold enough to confront me about my fat either. The only person who had done so was Gladys. She was the elderly woman at the phone survey job I had quit the month before, my only legacy a TV dinner forgotten in the refrigerator. Gladys worked in the booth next to me and had a son who was morbidly obese, so she took it upon herself to tell me that one of the reasons I couldn't find a better job even with my college degree was because people discriminated against morbidly obese people like me. Perhaps being old gave her more leeway to speak her mind, but I couldn't deny that she was right. It was amazing how many of my coworkers at that dead-end minimum wage job were obese. One woman looked like she'd had liposuction on her tummy and then regained weight. She looked like an upside-down mushroom with hips of bulging fat. Ironically, Gladys also offered me crackers and cookies during every shift. If she believed in nurturing with food, her son must have been well loved.

I was waiting for an intervention. Surely if I were drinking myself to death, someone would get my friends and family together, sit me down on the plaid couch in the family room for a good talking-to, and then send me off to a nicely landscaped facility for twenty-eight days. Why wasn't anyone ganging up on me because of my weight? I could guess it was only because weight is inexorably entwined with identity. Drinking and smoking are things that you do. Fat is something you are.

It was silly to wait for someone to fix me. I needed to fix myself. I knew what my problem was. I could no longer buy pants at the fat-girl store. And now, a doctor was offering weight-loss surgery as a serious option.

Weight-loss surgery. The "cure" for fatness.

It was the 99 percent guaranteed escape from morbid obesity. Thin chicks in infomercials may try to sell you diet pills as magical as Jack's beans or exercise devices that resemble alien machinery, but surgery is the real deal, no imitations or substitutions. You *will* become thinner. Or dead. Either way, it will change your life forever.

There are several types of weight-loss surgery. The kind my surgeon was pushing was called duodenal switch. To qualify for the surgery your body mass index had to be over forty (mine was over fifty).[1] It could also be lower if you had certain comorbidities. The word "comorbidities" sounds morbid in itself, but it refers to coexisting problems in addition to obesity, such as high blood pressure. The procedure reduces your stomach to the size of a baby's fist. Your small intestine is rerouted and shortened to inhibit the absorption of calories and nutrients. You have to take vitamins and drink protein shakes to prevent malnutrition. You can never eat a dozen donuts again without vomiting. Pop rocks and soda could actually make your stomach explode.

And you might die. Out of 16,155 cases studied in a 2005 article in the *Journal of the American Medical Association (JAMA)*, 2 percent of the patients studied died within thirty days of weight-loss surgery and 4.6 percent were dead within a year.[2] Many more suffer complications such as staple leaks, infections, and ulcers.[3] Risks decrease if you are younger and have an experienced surgeon, but the risks still exist.

A commercial for weight-loss surgery used to air frequently on my television. The sales pitch didn't focus on becoming thin but instead sold you the fabulous new life you would have once you became thin. Your wardrobe would contain only designer clothes. Suitors would duel with pistols over who could take you to The Olive Garden. Unicorns would follow you to work. You wouldn't just be thin; you would finally be happy and loved. The commercials sold you hope, just like the state lottery commission did. Buy a ticket and you too might become a millionaire. Rich, thin, either one would solve all your problems. It was all your dreams come true.

But what if it were a lie?

I knew thin people with perfect skin and perfectly miserable lives. It was easy to blame the fat for everything. It may be one reason I *stayed* fat. But could snipping and sewing my internal organs as if I were altering a dress really solve all my problems? Wasn't fat just as much a behavioral problem as a physical one? Was the threat of an exploding stomach really the only way to teach me discipline and follow-through?

The prospect of surgery was scary. I didn't consider it the easy way out. Brushing my teeth was easy; gastric surgery was not. I'd heard the stories. I didn't know what would be easy about endless phone calls with insurance company drones fighting to approve the procedure. Or recovering from surgery with plastic drains sticking out of my flesh that would make me look like a science fiction creation. Or taking pills for the rest of my life and drinking vile protein shakes that still might not prevent malnutrition. Or facing bouts of vomiting or diarrhea, code-named "dumping," if I ate two slices of cheesecake. I didn't know what would be easy about slicing through unblemished flesh, having my stomach rerouted so food permanently bypassed part of my intestines. It would be permanent construction on the highway of my gastric system. No exit ever again.

Not to mention the headtrip I'd be on after changing my body so drastically so quickly. Many weight-loss surgery patients reached their goal weight within a year. Scuba divers have to decompress slowly when moving from areas of high to low pressure. Going to sleep fat one year and waking up thin the next would probably give me a case of the bends in the brain.

When people said weight-loss surgery was the easy way out, they meant it was cheating. I don't consider life-saving medical procedures cheating, but not everyone agrees with me. If I had the surgery, I'd be physically changing my body so it would be nearly impossible for me to overeat without dire consequences. I would get thinner, but I would have to live with the implication that I didn't earn it in the same way as someone who ate cottage cheese and grapefruit and spent enough time on the Stairmaster to climb the Empire State Building. It certainly undermined the American dream that was hammered into me from youth, that if I worked hard enough and long enough I could do anything. If I lost weight via surgery there would always be the unspoken implication that I hadn't earned my thinness, that I hadn't done it the "right" way, that I would still be a weak and lazy fat person inside despite my smaller dress size.

I'd read blogs by people who'd considered the procedure or actually gone under the knife. They all recognized the gravity of the decision. It was heavier than I could ever be. In essence, I would be trading one set of health problems for another. Instead of heart disease or diabetes behind door A, I could choose dietary restrictions and possible malnutrition behind door B. I might also reach into the grab bag of horror stories: stitches bursting, leaking, abscesses, pulmonary embolism. It was the vocabulary of complications. The fact that people even considered undergoing such an extreme procedure was a testament to how much suffering morbid obesity could cause, mentally and physically.

There is another, less invasive form of weight loss surgery called adjustable gastric banding surgery. A silicone ring is inserted around your stomach to create a small pouch at the top, making you feel fuller faster. The band can be adjusted by filling it with saline. This surgery is gaining popularity, especially in Australia.[4] It was not yet popular in the United States at the time of my attack, and I was unaware of it as an option. I have no idea if I would have considered this procedure at the time, and I guess I never will.

I can only hope that a hundred years from now there will be better treatments for the severely overweight. I propose a virus that rewrites your brain cells to give you good exercise habits. It's sad that the only guaranteed method of weight loss available to me involved altering organs in my body to make them less efficient. There is something medieval about the procedure, a soul sister to the lobotomy. But what else is there? Is the cure worse than the disease? Disappointingly, most patients don't even become completely thin, just significantly less fat.[5] As many patients say, the surgery is just a tool, not a true cure.

I hope our fat descendants will laugh at the weight-loss treatments that are now in vogue. If people are still trying the grapefruit diet hundreds of years from now, God help us all. Nonetheless, I understood why people chose to have the surgery. Eventually the weight is just too much. You can't carry the load anymore, and not just in your joints. Ultimately, you do what you have to do. I wasn't going to judge anyone. One thin person wasn't superior to another just because one took the expressway and another took the scenic route. Most people spoke happily of the changes surgery had brought about in their lives, but I doubt a single one of them would have chosen it unless it was the absolute last resort.

Luckily I wasn't at my last resort. There were still several resorts on this highway—a Holiday Inn, a Days Inn, and a Motel 6 around the curve. On the ride home my mother and I talked.

"So," she said.

"Yeah," I replied. The dashboard rattled in time to the vibration from the engine as we waited at a red light.

"What are you thinking?" she said. I doubt she was any more eager than I was to have half my stomach removed. It's not as if I could sell it as tripe at the deli counter.

"I guess, after I have the gallbladder removed, I'll make a really serious effort to lose weight." I had never thrown myself completely gung-ho into an effort to become thinner. I couldn't let someone remove most of my stomach before I could honestly say I had tried everything else. "After a year, if that doesn't work . . . maybe then I'll start considering surgery."

This was the wake-up call I'd been waiting for. Lightning had struck. If I had been an alcoholic, I would have been on my way to rehab. If I had been a shopaholic, I would have been freezing my credit cards in blocks of ice in the freezer. I'd had my moment of clarity.

Only I didn't. I stayed fat for at least another year. Wake-up call received. Snooze button pushed.

I was wheeled into gallbladder surgery on a gurney. They put special pads around my legs that squeezed and released my legs like a massage. This was to prevent clotting, something I was at a higher risk for since I was so fat. I'm sure I must have paid extra for them, one more line item on the bill, hundreds of dollars farther away from paying off my credit card debt and enjoying a vacation in France.

I sat in bed in the pre-op room and tried to watch television. My mother tried distracting me with conversation. My mind couldn't focus on anything. This was a routine surgery with little risk, but people died during procedures as routine as face-lifts. There could be a fluke accident. I could die. This could be the end of the story of me and I'd never gotten around to writing it down. I was embarrassed that I'd let it come to this. If something went wrong, my life would come *only* to this.

Attendants wheeled my gurney down hallways, through double doors, and into the sterile operating room. I felt so vulnerable, lying on a rolling bed as nurses towered above me. I stared at unfamiliar ceilings. Fluorescent lights left dark shadowy impressions on my eyelids when I blinked.

I was conscious when I scooted from the gurney onto the operating table. I felt bad for the medical staff who would have to lift me back onto the gurney after surgery. Would the words "Shamu" or "Jabba the Hutt" be bandied about in jest? What did people use for fat metaphors before Sea World and George Lucas? Would my unconscious mind be able to remember their comedy selections when I awakened in the recovery room? I should have hidden a recording device up my ass. Obesity made me paranoid about what everyone thought of me, but was it paranoia if it turned out to be true?

The anesthesiologist stood by my right side and asked me to give him my arm.

"What will this feel like?" I asked him, focusing only on the pair of eyes peeking out over the surgical mask. I can't remember if they were blue or green or brown.

"I don't know. No one's ever told me before."

He inserted the needle into my IV.

"Oh, it's like a muscle cramp in my arm. It feels kind of—"

Then I was staring at another unfamiliar ceiling, waking up in recovery.

One advantage of having the surgery so young was that I recovered quickly. I didn't just bounce back, I ricocheted off the walls. My weight loss was off to a great start. I had lost several ounces when my gallstones and organ tissue were pitched into a biohazard waste bin. When I looked at superthin supermodels in magazines, I wondered how they could possibly cram all their internal organs and bones into the slender envelope of their skin. Could there be a secret supermodel organ donation cabal?

There's never a good time for surgery, but the timing was particularly terrible for me because I had gotten a real job as a web developer only a week before my attack. I was still on my college's severely inadequate health insurance plan. After surgery, I threw billing statements back and forth with the HMO for more than six months, which I magnanimously refrained from folding into deadly ninja stars. Ultimately I ended up paying 70 percent of the total bill. You can make money by selling a kidney, so why did I have to pay so much to have this particular organ removed? My dreams of LASIK surgery, a shiny new car, and a trip to Europe would have to remain a byproduct of REM sleep. I was doomed to be a blind homebody whose car rendered abstract art on the garage floor with transmission fluid.

A blind, *fat* homebody.

CHAPTER 4

No Epiphanies

I kept my promise about losing weight . . . at first. The fear of death was fresh and the scars still pink and raised above my skin. I didn't want to put my family through the affair of tracking down an extra-wide coffin. I was filled with hopeful trepidation This could be it. For real. The start of a remarkable transformation that would completely redefine how others would see me. I took the "before" picture.

I called a local gym and got a quote on what it would cost to join. Then I hung up and called the YMCA. Then I hung up and decided to walk around the block.

I started a food diary, which, like all of my previous diaries, was abandoned after three days. The only thing more boring than writing down every item of food I'd eaten was reading every item of food I'd eaten. It was supposed to shock me into realizing I was consuming the gross national product of Ecuador daily. Mostly it just made me crazy trying to remember if I'd had a soda with lunch. I started a secret weight-loss blog. No one read that either.

After two days I fell off the wagon and into the chocolate stash in my bottom desk drawer. There were chocolate Riesen and mint chocolate cups hidden behind my file folders of credit card statements and medical bills, forming a diorama of cause and effect. I hadn't trashed the candy because I thought it would be wasteful to throw out food. My parents had never made me clean my plate as a child and they'd never lectured me about starving kids in Ethiopia, but it seemed wrong to throw out something edible instead of eating it. Food didn't grow on trees . . . except when it did. I had to find my chocolate bars a good home, like placing unwanted cats or puppies.

This was, of course, ridiculous.

There are not homeless people lurking outside fat girls' kitchens waiting to devour unwanted baked goods. I wasn't running a bundt cake relocation program. My brother had worked in the fast-food industry, and the amount of burgers and fries they tossed out at the end of the day was worse than a year's worth of my food-wasting sins.

After three days, I stopped updating the blog. When it comes to weight-loss blogs, no news is bad news. My next entry came in March, when I confessed I'd fallen off the wagon again. One day we will all drive flying cars, and people will still be falling off wagons. My impetus to hop back on was a pain in my chest, near my heart. I had lain in bed the night before, cat curled under my knees, wondering if I would embody the lyrics of Y Kant Tori Read's song and have a heart attack at twenty-three. Obesity caused so many aches and pains that I was a hypochondriac, constantly trying to convince myself I wasn't dying of heart disease or cancer, or that I didn't need a new knee. After the bill for my surgery, I couldn't afford a replacement knee, but mine had started creaking, especially on the walk downstairs from my fourth-floor office.

My mother bought a treadmill and a smoothie blender. I started parking farther away in parking lots to sneak more exercise into my day. I bought a green lacy top a size too small as motivation to stick with the program.

I lasted four days that time. If I kept lasting one more day on each attempt, I might be thin by the time those flying cars appeared.

At the end of April, I posted only one entry. It denounced the grocery store designers who placed Krispy Kreme glazed donuts at the entrance of the store, as if that were my real problem.

I tried a third time in July. I had learned that taking the stairs every day could lead to an extra five pounds of weight loss a year. Little spurts of calorie usage here and there added up through time, just like the fistful of spare change my father would dump into an old check box on his dresser every day after work. Once the box was full, we'd dump it out and sort the coins into paper rolls. We'd end up with tens of dollars in the shapes of brown cylinders to exchange for cash. I would gather up my weight in the same way and exchange it for a better body.

When I descended the stairs at the end of the day, I stopped short at a pain in my right joint. I had to hobble down the six flights of stairs, taking baby steps, landing two feet on each step before descending to the next. How was I going to lose weight if my body wouldn't cooperate with the simplest of exercises?

In October I gave up soda. In November I took it back.

Later in November I ordered a scale that measured up to 440 pounds. I don't know why I'd tried to lose weight without owning one. It was foolhardy when I couldn't tell how much I'd lost. My reckoning arrived in a big, brown cardboard box. Numbers are normally such cold and expressionless digits when posted on price tags or written on calendars, but they seemed so warm and encouraging when they told me how much I had achieved in a week.

I pulled it out of the box and inserted two AA batteries into the back. I stepped on the scale until it went BEEP, BEEP, indicating it was done judging me, as opposed to most people, who only silently judged me. I hesitantly peeked at the number between my toes.

368.8 pounds.

I was relieved I hadn't rolled my weight odometer over into the four hundreds. I felt as if I'd lost thirty pounds simply by stepping on the scale's white plastic frame. I swore that these digits would be going down.

Looking back at those early blog entries, I can see I was confident and full of hope, yet I sit here in the future like Cassandra, knowing I was doomed. It's like reading a book I already know the ending to. "Silly girl! You're not going to escape from the dungeon until chapter five. Didn't you get the revised copy of the text?"

Perhaps as you're reading this you're wondering, "When's it going to happen? When's she going to start losing weight for real?"

I wanted to know too.

I thought about giving up.

I might not be capable of being thin. I might be like a no-talent actress who should blow off auditions and drive my beat-up Chevrolet home from L.A. I typically scoffed at destiny. It's a force that controls characters in fantasy novels, not real people like me without pointy ears who own only magic wands made by Hitachi. But "destiny" is the only word that described how I felt about my fat in my most fatalistic moments.

Even if I did lose the weight, I had heard most people regained it. If I were to call the customer support number of any major dieting corporation for its rates of recidivism, I knew I wouldn't get them. I had better odds in Vegas, and at least the food at casinos was free. I could just be grateful that I lived in a society in which food was plentiful enough for me to become so fat. Obesity was surely better than emaciation.

Was thin even something I should want? I wanted to be considered attractive by the average male, but I didn't want to define myself only by my relationship to men. I wanted to find clothes more easily, but retailers seemed partly to blame for ignoring a steadily growing portion of the population. I wanted to feel comfortable in a crowd and unashamed of myself when meeting new people, but that might be a mental problem I needed to overcome, not a physical one.

The fat-acceptance movement had a lot to say about this topic. I was traipsing along the Internet, throwing stones into cyberspace, when I heard about organizations such as the National Association to Advance Fat Acceptance (NAAFA). I clicked on websites that preached that fat people should accept themselves at the size they were and that society should accept that not everyone could be thin. They fought fat discrimination and declared that the diet industry did more harm than good. There was even a group of plus-size cheerleaders flashing the cellulite on their chubby legs beneath short black skirts. Joining the synchronized swimming group was out of the question, though. I could barely even dog-paddle.

I cruised a lot of these websites, burning a fraction of a calorie with each mouse click, trying to get a better sense of the movement as a whole. There were interesting discussions about whether the health consequences of obesity were exaggerated because of a moral panic.[1] The moderates seemed reasonable enough when they argued that you could be fat and fit. Plenty of chubby people finished marathons every year. But I didn't believe that meant all fat people were healthy either, especially the fatter they got. I couldn't gauge the cholesterol level of the 500-pound woman at the grocery store just by looking at her, but I *could* see that she had to use a motorized scooter because she couldn't walk. She didn't seem to be a paragon of health. There was a point at which fat no longer seemed like something to be accepted but a matter of life and death.

There was a difference between being forty pounds overweight and being 400 pounds. If you got flesh-eating gangrene because you couldn't clean your ass properly, you had a problem. If you were so overweight that you stopped breathing while you slept, you definitely had a problem. And you'd wish you had either one of those problems if your toes were chopped off, not to fit into Cinderella's slipper and fool a prince, but because they had turned black and rotted off from diabetes. None of the sites I visited talked about this. For a movement that was about acceptance, there appeared to be some denial going on.

I liked the idea of equal rights and self-esteem at any size. I wanted to be paid the same as my thin counterparts, but statistics showed that was unlikely to happen.[2] I certainly wanted to like my body as much as the obese burlesque troupe seemed to like theirs, though I wasn't sure where I could find a pair of fishnet stockings in my size. Its members didn't seem ashamed of being fat. I'd never seen that before. I didn't even know that was possible.

I bookmarked some of the fat-acceptance sites, but I still wanted to lose weight. This did not go over well. One day I logged into my account on a fat-acceptance message board to leave a comment and discovered I was not allowed to post. At first I assumed this was because Internet gremlins had caused an error while munching on the server's motherboards. Later, I learned it was because weight-loss bloggers were not allowed on that site. It turned out this was detailed in the registration agreement, which I had scrolled through quickly without reading when I'd created my account. I should really start reading those things before I accidentally sign away my firstborn child, assuming I haven't already.

Fine. I wasn't paying the server bills; I didn't get to make the rules. Still, I was pissed. I weighed more than most of those people. I hated fat bigotry as much as any of them. I had never even been on a diet like many of them. But my voice would no longer be heard because I wanted to be thin. Why was that such a problem? I wasn't trying to convince anyone else to lose a couple of pounds. Weight was such a personal issue that I hadn't even talked to my family about it. I couldn't imagine telling a stranger on the Internet that he or she needed to lose weight. But neither could I honestly say that I was happy that I lost my breath when I tossed a ball around with the cat. Walking down the hallway and picking up a jingling ball three times shouldn't be a workout.

The definition of the word acceptance is "to recognize as true." Acceptance is the opposite of denial. If I really accepted myself as I was, it meant I'd recognized who I was to the best of my ability, flaws and all. It didn't mean I was necessarily satisfied with all the materials that made the house of me. The kitchen tile needed to be replaced, the patio door was squeaking, and what *was* I thinking when I chose that wallpaper? But at least I'd taken a look around the place and written an honest appraisal. It didn't mean I couldn't hire a contractor. The house of me had a strong foundation, but I wanted to paint the walls a different color and add a Jacuzzi.

Just because I'd accepted who I was didn't mean I had to cryogenically freeze myself as that person for the rest of my life. If I were the same person twenty years from now, I would have wasted my life as an organic air recycler. Acceptance did not equal complacency. I didn't have to throw up my hands and say, "Okay! This is it. This is as good as it gets." I could accept myself and be working to change myself at the same time. I knew it would be only when I truly accepted myself that real change would be possible.

However, I would not be able to change myself into someone with posting access to this message board. After my account was deleted, it was clear I wasn't wanted, so I stopped visiting the site. I believed people shouldn't hate themselves for being overweight, but I didn't think they should have to enjoy it either. I had accepted that I was fat. I just couldn't *like* being fat. It wasn't because I hated myself, an accusation some fat-acceptance members frequently threw at dieters. I wanted to lose weight because I loved myself and I knew I deserved better.

I think the site's attitude was just a reaction to the poor way fat people are treated. Some thin people who'd never battled a weight problem assumed I was simply weak willed, that if I just laid off the Twinkies I wouldn't be so fat. These were stereotypes used by people trying to oversimplify the issue. Fat was not a moral problem. It was a complex state caused by too many factors to name. I think the FA members got tired of being blamed for being fat when it wasn't completely under their control. They didn't like to be called lazy when they'd worked for years on diets that didn't work. And even if I had been the laziest, weakest-willed person on the planet, being fat did not make me a bad person. Fat wasn't good or bad. It wasn't a scarlet F of shame written on my elbow. It was just fat. I deserved as much respect as any thin person and I shouldn't have to live under a cloud of shame.

The antidote to shame is pride, but I thought some FA members took the pride so far that they were creating shame in the other direction, in an equal and opposite reaction. Whenever I tried hanging around fat-acceptance sites, I felt as if they were trying to make me feel bad for wanting to be thin, which was just as bad as anyone who tried to make me feel bad for being fat. Just because you believed fat was good didn't mean thin was necessarily bad. There were certainly many bad things that came from the importance society put on being slender: anorexia, bulimia, and a diet industry that made millions of dollars without making millions of customers thinner. If society put importance on being fat there would be a different list of bad things: binge eating, forced feedings, and poorer gas mileage. Either way, there were many things about being fat that simply sucked, my surgery bill being one of them. My knees had only so much cartilage left.

I also had the nagging feeling that this was about more than just fat and thin. It was about a philosophy toward life. The members of the fat-acceptance movement were encouraging me to give up hope of ever being smaller. It was as though they had decided I'd be locked away in fat prison forever, so I should just hang some drapes over the steel bars to make the place homey. My body *was* like a prison, isolating me from relationships and experiences that I so desperately wanted. I kept hearing the subliminal message, "Stop trying. You'll never make it. Forget about digging an escape tunnel. It'll just add six more months to your sentence." Underlying all the adipose tissue was a philosophical debate greater than fat or thin, pretty or ugly. It was the battle of whether it was better to strive for the impossible dream or to settle for what I had. Which one would cause more casualties?

Many fat-acceptance members believed obesity wasn't a choice but a permanent life sentence handed down by your genetics and metabolism. After reading the most recent research, I agreed that it was much harder for some people to lose weight than others.[3] Factors you had little control over could make you fatter. People struggling to get by couldn't afford the lean meats and fresh vegetables that the middle class could.[4] Some people seemed to gain weight if they ate half a cookie, while others couldn't bulk up no matter how much cake they ate. Some scientists speculated obesity could even be caused by a virus.[5] None of this was fair, and it created a very uneven playing field, but that didn't mean it was impossible to lose weight. Deciding it wasn't a choice sounded like a choice itself.

Simply believing you could do something was essential for success. The placebo effect is well documented. If you give sick people a pill they believe will make them better, it will usually improve their health even if they're just chewing on a Mentos. In one study, girls who took a math test after being told boys were better at math scored worse than girls who didn't hear this information.[6] The very act of believing you couldn't do something made it less likely that you could. It was a self-fulfilling prophecy.

If there were simply a self-acceptance movement, maybe I could have joined that.

The rebukes I got from FA members for wanting to lose weight were strikingly similar in tone to the criticisms fat people got for being fat. In both instances people claimed to be criticizing me for my own good and wanted to know why I couldn't see the error of my ways; they just couldn't agree on what the error was, getting fat or trying to get thin. The members of the FA movement were promoting what they thought was the best life philosophy for fat people, but I also knew that it would really piss them off if I lost 200 pounds and kept it off for the rest of my life. Many of these people truly believed that fat people could never permanently lose weight. If I did it anyway it would strike a blow to their personal philosophy. While they probably believed getting me to give up before I even tried was in my best interests, it was also in their best interests to defend the worldview they depended upon to keep themselves sane. I didn't need them to look out for my own good. I didn't like being told what I could or couldn't do. I didn't want to give up.

I liked the FA movement best when it was promoting things I hadn't believed to be possible, like wearing a bathing suit in public without being ashamed. I wanted to continue focusing on possibilities, not limitations. I wanted to be a medium in an average-size world. I wanted to cross my legs and hook one ankle behind the other. I wanted to feel my collarbones. I wanted to live in a country without crash dieting, where people didn't hate themselves for their size, be it fat, thin, or shifting in between.

When I finally accepted myself, I accepted that I didn't want to be fat. And that was okay.

I wasn't the only one who didn't want to buy shirts with the word "extra-large" on the tag. My younger brother, Jim, was waging a war on fat. When he ran on the treadmill the basement door would rattle on its hinges in fear of the oncoming campaign. He'd constructed a barrier on the top of our refrigerator with large plastic powder bottles featuring bodybuilders on the labels. My long neglected smoothie blender was conscripted to mix creatine shakes.

And he lost weight. He beat back the army of fat cells, carved out a spot in the enemy lines, and held his ground. He wanted to draft me to join the fray too.

It must have been hard for my family to see me get so big, and not just because I took up more space on the couch when we were watching TV. If I were worried about me, they must have been too, but I didn't want to talk about it. Talking about something made it real. I had now become the fattest person in the family, but I kept the topic off-limits.

One night I was channel surfing when I caught part of the reality show *The Biggest Loser*, on which people competed to lose weight. It was unusual to see fat people on television. Overweight people get a lot of shit about watching too much TV, but fat people are rarely ever cast on shows. When *The Sopranos* went off the air, the percentage of fat actors on television must have been cut in half. I especially hated it when a thin actor wore a fat suit. It felt like the fat version of blackface. We got to laugh at all the stupid stereotypes the actor was portraying without having to feel bad about laughing at an actual fat person. I was curious to watch these reality show contestants playing out my fantasies at the fat farm. It seemed as if most of them wanted to lose weight more than they wanted to win the money. Thin was the real prize, not the cash.

When I heard the sound of rubber soles on parquet floor, I clicked the button for the next channel on the remote faster than if I were ringing in on *Jeopardy!* I didn't want to be caught watching shows about fat people for the same reason I didn't wear a T-shirt that said, "Ask me about my obesity problem."

But they noticed anyway, the caring, concerned bastards. Jim would go on and on about the diet he was on. I'd walk into the kitchen and inhale the strawberry dust cloud of powdered protein milk shake, becoming a victim of second-hand shake. He'd mumble something about insulin levels and the evils of white flour. I'd chomp on garlic and onion bagels with the confused look of a cat being lectured on thermodynamics. He'd talk about the benefits of whole grains and vegetables and I'd wonder if there were such a thing as a half grain.

He was simply excited to share his new knowledge. He never called me fat, and he never pressured me to go on a diet. He just left the diet book lying around and walked around eighty pounds thinner.

It was really annoying.

He was, after all, the same person who introduced me to the dollar menu at McDonald's. At least I knew he genuinely cared about my health and not just my looks. I'd often heard people say that I should lose weight because it was unhealthy, but coming from strangers it seemed like the politically correct way of saying, "Fat people are disgusting." The health thing was just a handy coincidence. There are many other unhealthy habits that don't have the social stigma that obesity does. Stress and lack of sleep are bad for you, but people who work eighty-hour weeks and sleep four hours a night are often applauded for their work ethic, not denounced for weakening their immune systems.[7] I sometimes asked strangers not to smoke around me, but it wasn't because I cared about their future visits to the oncology ward. I just didn't like inhaling the fog of someone's cigarette smoke. I doubt everyone who told me fat was unhealthy genuinely cared about my risk for heart disease. If people wanted a better view than what I was providing, they could buy a house in the Hamptons.

I was hesitant to try Jim's plan, though. My diet prejudice was still in full effect. I believed you could eat healthily, but I was suspicious of anything that came packaged in a book or could be labeled a "fad." It was the end of 2004 and we were at the peak of the low-carb craze, a time when you could order a double cheeseburger without the bun and the cashier wouldn't blink. But I didn't have much left to lose. Actually, I had a lot to lose. That was the problem. I was willing to consider extreme options like dieting.

Yet I was still afraid of being gullible or wrong. I hated being wrong. I didn't want to try something that would later be shown to be absurd and ineffective. I didn't want to hear, "You tried the Tapeworm Diet? Did you replace all your brain cells with fat cells?" I was already fat. I didn't want to be stupid too. I didn't want to endanger my health either. Ironic, yes, but I didn't want to trade my obesity problems for crazy dieting problems.

But Jim was thinner and not crazy as far as I knew. He wasn't eating raw leeches for breakfast. He didn't consume only blue foods on Fridays. He wasn't drinking raw eggs in the morning and running fifty miles a day. But as a twenty year old he *had* read that a human male reached his physical peak at twenty-one and muttered, "Oh, crap." Then he did something about it.

The diet book sat on my desk for a couple of weeks near the end of the year. I decided it would be as pointless to start a diet during the holiday bingeing season as it was to shovel the driveway while it was snowing. Even though I devoured chocolate-covered cherries and sugar cookies during Christmas, I amazingly weighed the same 372 pounds as I had before Thanksgiving. I hadn't even been exercising.

I read the book before the end of the year. It didn't tell me exactly what carbohydrates were, but I had a much better picture of how my body processed them. I finally learned why diabetes made you blind and caused your toes to fall off. Mostly I learned about the intricacies of the dance between my food and my body, steps I should have learned years ago but that were never covered in health class.

The new year came. Noisemakers officially sounding off the beginning of the dieting season. On my blog I posted this on January 13, 2005.

> *Enough.*
> *Oh really, let's just fucking do this already! Here. Now. No more waiting.*

Another in a long line of bold statements. It had many older sisters and cousins. This time it even included profanity. It was different only because this time it was true.

There are lots of ways to measure weight-loss progress. I took my measurements, but I didn't know how accurate they were since I never seemed to get the same number twice. My sixty-inch tape measure couldn't fit all the way around my hips anyway. In high school gym class my coach had demonstrated a method of measuring body fat by using calipers to measure several points on the body. I didn't know where I could find someone to do that nor did I want a stranger fondling my underarm fat. There are some scales that will estimate your body weight by sending an undetectable electrical pulse through your feet. I couldn't find one that would weigh people of more than 330 pounds.

I had heard one of the most accurate ways to determine someone's body fat was to weigh him or her underwater. Fat was buoyant, so you could calculate your body composition based on the measurements. I was offered the opportunity to be weighed this way as extra credit for a college psychology class (the researchers were always looking for coeds to experiment on), but I didn't volunteer. I couldn't imagine myself floating around naked in a tank for a bunch of scientists in lab coats. I would have felt like a polar bear swimming by the glass observation area at the zoo. The only way I could weigh myself like that at home would be if I stole the lobster tank from the grocery store. Even if I figured out how to sneak it out of the store, I'd still have to scrub it clean of lobster poop.

I decided to stick to the bathroom scale to track my progress. It measured only my gravitational attraction to the earth, not my levels of fat and lean muscle mass, but it was easy to use and objective. I could also plug my weight and height into a formula to determine my body mass index. A BMI under 18.5 is considered underweight, 18.5 to 25 is normal, 25-30 is overweight, 30 and above is obese. The BMI was developed in the mid-1800s by Adolphe Quetelet as a tool to determine people's ideal weight based on statistical data.[8] Insurance companies started using it to help ascertain the risk of insuring clients. Its medical relevance is questionable, unless you're comfortable letting your statistician or insurance adjuster handle your medical procedures. I certainly felt as if I'd had a colonoscopy after I saw my latest auto policy rates. The BMI is somewhat flawed since it categorizes muscular athletes like Shaquille O'Neal as obese. I understood it wasn't perfect, but I found it handy to get a general sense of what weight range I should be aiming for. In college I'd set my goal weight to 140, but if I were under 169 my BMI would be "normal," so I decided to loosen my standards for thinness. I was also working as an independent contractor, so BMI mattered a lot when I unsuccessfully applied for a personal health insurance policy. The more likely you were to actually use health insurance, the more likely you were to be denied it.

Being overweight was like being in debt. Instead of owing money, I owed calories. I arbitrarily set my goal weight at 160, a number that would set my body mass index as normal but wasn't so low that it seemed unattainable. It also ended in a zero. There was an unspoken law that your goal weight had to end in a zero or a five.

It takes approximately 3,500 calories to burn a pound of fat. Multiply that by 212 pounds to lose and I was 742,000 calories overdrawn. My body was charging interest via my disintegrating health. I could hear it when my knees creaked and see it in those little pink scars from my surgery.

A 24-year-old woman who weighs 160 pounds and engages in light activity will burn about 2,200 calories a day, give or take. Divide 742,000 by 2,200 and you'll find I was about 337 days ahead on my eating. Essentially, I'd eaten almost a year's worth of food that I hadn't needed to. I was overdrawn and overweight.

The math is a bit more complicated than that, of course. As I got larger I needed more calories to sustain my weight, so I shouldn't technically count that as excess. To properly figure out how many calories overdrawn I was, I'd have to remember how to do calculus, which I don't because I never thought it would have any practical application in my life. If my precalculus book had included word problems about fat girls, I probably would have changed my mind.

It's not surprising that I had credit card debt as well. Twelve cavities and a broken transmission had been bad for my credit rating. Solving both problems demanded similar approaches. I had to figure out what I owed, pay down a little at a time, and chart my goals and progress. I needed to catch up on my exercise payments. Flossing would be a good idea too.

On January 15, 2005, I started walking again because that's what I always did. It seemed quaint to start the journey of a thousand miles with one step. At my size there weren't many other options. You're probably wondering what diet I followed too. I'm not going to tell you. There are plenty of books that will be happy to tell you what to eat. There isn't one diet to rule them all. Atkins, South Beach, Weight Watchers—you'll find people who've lost hundreds of pounds on any of them. Typically their results are not typical. I did research, compared options, and eventually settled on something that could fit into my life. It was something I could see myself doing forever without hating my existence.

On February 6, 2005, I wrote in my blog:

> *I am feeling really good about myself. I know that this time I am actually going to go all the way and lose the weight. I've started thinking about things I'll do when I'm skinny, not "if" I were skinny.*

I started plowing down through the numbers, leaving decimals and fractions in my wake. I checked my scalp. My hairs weren't sticking out on end. Lightning had not struck me in a thunderclap of epiphany. There was no moment of revelation, no burning bush. There was no sign from God. But I was on my way.

This was it, *for real.*

CHAPTER 5

Diet and Exercise

It would have been simplest if I could just stop eating. I wanted to tell my body to switch to backup power and burn those fat cells instead of demanding more food. I could pop a multivitamin a day to ward off scurvy. I'd hibernate in the woods with the bears all winter, wrapped in a coat of fat that would melt off my bones by the springtime. Instead, my only realistic option was to consume fewer calories than I burned. I hoped I wouldn't find myself holding up the local Krispy Kreme in a sugar-crash psychosis, wielding a grapefruit spoon like a shiv.

I needed to eat healthy, but what did that mean? Would I have to consume only locally grown organic foods? Become a vegan? Give up carbohydrates? What exactly was a carbohydrate besides the latest health buzz word? And how was I going to learn all this without adding "registered dietician" to my resume?

Figuring out what was healthy seemed as subjective as determining who was the prettiest girl in a beauty pageant, but I had to start somewhere, even if there were flaws in the concepts I'd learned. If I kept doing what I was doing, I'd keep getting what I always got—fat.

I started with the diet book my brother had found helpful, hoping the publisher wouldn't issue a revised copy the next year recalling the previous advice.

Thankfully the book didn't refer to foods as "good" and "bad," as though we could assign philosophical concepts of morality to the items we eat. There wasn't a "wrong" way to eat either, except if you tried stuffing cheeseburgers up your ass. It did list certain foods to enjoy and others to avoid. I copied down a list of items that weren't up for arraignment in food court and got in my car, saying a silent thank-you to Oldsmobile for its extra-long seat belts.

Then I drove to McDonald's.

Before I started this healthy-eating nonsense, I was going to have a "farewell to junk food" bash. I ordered a Big Mac, large fries, and a soda so large that it barely fit in my cup holder. I drove back home and ate every piece of my meal, even the lettuce that fell into small puddles of mayonnaise on the plastic wrapper. Feeling full, I got back into my car and headed for the grocery store. I wasn't supposed to shop on an empty stomach anyway.

I waddled through the automated sliding doors and avoided looking at my image in the closed-circuit security monitors. The official greeter welcomed me to the store as I quickly grabbed a cart. I stopped at the red tile that marked the beginning of the produce section. I had not spent much time among the radishes and rutabagas in the few years I'd shopped for my own groceries. If someone removed all the stickers labeling items, I wouldn't have been able to identify 40 percent of the produce. What were those funny white bulbs with stalks of hair messier than my own? What should I call the long green vegetables in the next bin that were thinner than I'd ever be? Like a substitute teacher, I didn't know any names.

I wasn't sure if I should buy new foods or just stick to the vegetables that I could name. I walked up and down the aisles, avoiding the misty jets of water that kept the celery fresh. I leaned over to strangle a head of broccoli when my eyes beheld the pastry section nestled in an alcove behind the rows of lettuce. Croissants, cookies, and coconut cake, oh my. I needed to get out of there before I did something stupid. I pushed my weight behind the left side of the cart to make a sharp right turn and dashed to the safety of the dairy section, though my dash was more like a slow jog.

The cheese aisle wasn't any easier to navigate. I appreciated the variety of culinary choices available since I had no desire to eat grits every day like my Depression-era ancestors. However, I had no idea if I needed low-fat cheese, fat-free cheese, or cheese made from part-skim milk. Did all these varieties even taste like cheese, or was I buying a synthetic cheeselike compound that was created in a lab next to a vat of Silly Putty?

I grabbed two tubs of different types of ricotta, comparing the nutritional information on the back, only partially understanding what the numbers and percentages meant. They made as much sense as the Spanish soap operas on cable. My smattering of substandard Spanish classes in middle school had never explained why the maid was slapping the priest in the confessional booth. Protein, sodium, calories from fat—all of this surely meant something, but I didn't know what.

A gray-haired woman with a perm knocked her cart into mine. I was inhibiting the trade of curd-based substances by blocking access to the shredded mozzarella. I randomly picked a tub of ricotta and moved on. Tempted to grab a cylinder of potato chips in a cardboard display case at the end of an aisle, I stepped up the pace. My exercise plan so far consisted of running away from food. If I hired one of the stock boys to chase me around the store with a licorice whip, I'd be thin by Christmas.

As long as I stuck to the edges of the building, I could avoid most temptations. The produce, dairy, and meat sections were safe zones that lined the outer boundaries of the store. I tempted fate when I darted into the aisles where the packaged cookies dwelled. I made one or two swoops into the aisles to get diet sodas and sugar-free gelatin. I wanted to head for the candy section out of habit. I had always loved grabbing a box of Junior Mints and chomping on them on the ride home. Today the only thing I'd be chewing on in the car was my fingernails. Picking out healthy food was like taking a pop quiz in nutrition that I hadn't studied hard enough for. Fearful that the Toll House elves might toss a bag of cookies into my cart if I lingered too long, I headed to the checkout line.

Fat-free yogurt, string cheese, and Lean Cuisines rolled down the conveyor belt ahead of me. I felt as if I were buying someone else's groceries. For the first time, I wasn't worried that the cashier would silently judge my purchases, unlike the time I bought a can of frosting purely for the purpose of eating it off a spoon. A junkie might need a spoon, heroin, and a lighter to get a fix, but I had substituted white powder with buttercream to mainline sugar. I had created an elaborate story to tell the cashier if she gave me a judgmental glance. "I have a sister, a skinny sister of course, so it's okay for her to be eating junk, and I just finished baking her a chocolate birthday cake (double-layered chocolate fudge, *Betty Crocker* cookbook, page 126) when I realized I didn't have powdered sugar, and since I had to go to the grocery store anyway, I decided to get the premade frosting, which I will now take directly home and smother on her cake with a spatula."

This was also the same imaginary party for which I was buying a dozen two liters of soda when they were on sale. But my elaborate backstories never stopped the cashier from swiping the bar code over the mean red lines of the scanner while jokingly saying, "You must be really thirsty."

I paid the cashier, returned home, and carried my numerous plastic bags into the kitchen. I was prepared for eating healthy or surviving the

Apocalypse. I opened the refrigerator to store my scavenged goods; a spatial dimensions IQ test ensued, rearranging everything to fit.

The kitchen counter wasn't any better. Astronomers discovered the existence of Pluto only because of its gravitational effects on other planets. I knew we had a kitchen counter because all those papers and dishes had to be resting on something. In a gesture of support, my mother cleared the section of the counter between the light switch and the sink for me, so I would have somewhere to cook. Now I wouldn't have to relocate stacks of paper and coffee stained mugs before figuring out what to do with all these vegetables I'd bought. I didn't even like vegetables.

I liked to eat food, but I didn't like to make it. Cooking was a task I left to my roommates or the teenage wage slave at the pizza delivery joint. I'd learned some basic cooking skills from my mom, but the most complicated meals I'd made included shaking and baking or grilling cheese. Many nights my meals were prepared simply by hitting the "Start" button on the microwave. Amazingly, this was more culinary education than some people got. One summer I brought the girl I babysat over to my house to play a video game. As we walked through the kitchen her eyes widened at the sight of brownies in an old scratched silver pan on the counter.

"Did your mom *make* those?" she asked in wonder.

"Yeah," I said, slightly confused. Had she never seen brownies before? Then I realized everything I'd prepared at her house came prepackaged in plastic and cardboard. She seemed unaware that you could prepare food using eggs and flour and sugar instead of pushing a tray into a microwave. Her mother was a single working mom, so I couldn't blame her for not serving a ten layer lasagna every night. Who had the time for that? Not me.

I never planned what I was going to eat until I was hungry, which was like waiting until I was drunk to start driving. As a child I would bang the cupboard doors open and closed, pushing aside cans of baking soda or shortening, searching for something to satiate my appetite instantly. Sometimes I'd discover a Carmello bar hidden behind the saltines. When I saw squirrels digging up nuts in the backyard, I wondered how many pounds of chocolate were hidden in drawers and cupboards and closets in our home at one time. Typically I would slam the final cupboard door closed and yell, "There's nothing to eat!" as if we lived in a model home stocked with Styrofoam fruit. My mother would ask us to add items we wanted to the grocery list, but I could never think of anything to write down.

I didn't have a spouse with whom to trade sexual favors for a hot dinner. I couldn't hire a chef to cook all my food. And no amount of bribery was going to get my roommates to cook for me every night. I couldn't afford to eat out every night, either. That would be difficult to do anyway since the healthiest item on most fast-food restaurants' menus was a wilted salad, and restaurant portions were usually gargantuan; today's small beverage cup was yesterday's large. I always overate when I was given big servings.

It was inevitable: I would have to learn how to cook. The best way to control what I ate was to prepare it myself. This was going to be painful, literally. My feet began to hurt if I stood for more than five minutes, but if I could survive a nine-hour gallbladder attack, I could withstand bowing arches after ten minutes in front of a skillet.

My diet book had some recipes in the back, but they included strange ingredients like "shallots" and "littleneck clams." I didn't even know clams had necks. I started a search for recipes online and nixed anything too complex. Anything that involved separating egg whites or getting out the sifter was a no-go. I wasn't even sure we owned a flour sifter. I also had zero tolerance for weird ingredients. I was not averse to buying one or two new spices or veggies for a recipe, but if it turned into a grocery store scavenger hunt that required me to find eye of newt, it was out. No toil or trouble.

I bought a recipe book that had "15-Minute Recipes" in the title. I found quick and easy recipes on Internet message boards. I mutilated enough vegetables with my poor knife skills to fill a mass grave, but as with any skill, the more I practiced the better I got. I figured out how to slice a tomato without slicing off my thumbs, though the red gooey insides did resemble blood. I collected six or seven quick recipes that didn't make me curse my sense of taste. It was repetitive, but it was safe. I wasn't feeling adventurous; I just wanted something that worked.

I envied my younger brother, who was a food freestyle master. I once watched him season some pork chops with a random assortment of spices and toss them in a skillet with some canned tomatoes for pizzazz and hope it would be edible when the sauces stopped sizzling. I preferred to have directions with precise measurements, specific cooking lengths, and tastiness ensured. If I were going to spend all that time chopping and mixing, I wanted to be pouring the result down my throat, not down the garbage disposal.

By summer, cooking became normal to me. It wasn't enjoyable, but it was a tolerable part of my day, like the half-hour commute to work. There is comfort in the familiar, even if the familiar is painful. I was being indoctrinated.

I was surprised that the food tasted good. I'd always thought of healthy food as bland, ill-tasting mush manufactured out of soybeans. Diet foods were marketed as having no fats, no sugars, and no carbs— all the stuff that tasted good. Yet now I was eating healthier without scraping the taste buds off my tongue with a spork after every meal.

I started wearing down the linoleum on my shopping route through the grocery store after only a month. Good choices became easier to make and I experienced significantly less terror among the cheese wheels. I realized my new approach to eating had reached my subconscious when I yelled at someone in a dream for daring to offer me a bowl of white rice. Any concerns that dream might have raised about my state of mind were outweighed by the feeling of empowerment I got when I passed pints of ice cream without opening the freezer door. While I wasn't anorexic or bulimic, I started to understand why women with eating disorders said they liked the control it gave them over their lives.

Surprisingly, I didn't miss candy and chips and cookies that much. Once I stopped eating them I stopped craving them. I'd spent the first week without them in a light-headed, low-carb daze, fixated on the moment after my induction period when I'd finally be able to eat an apple. But once the junk food was out of my life, I saw how bad our relationship together had been, and I was glad we'd broken up. I still missed fast food. Not the food, just the fast part. I was always planning now, more prepared than any Boy Scout. I predicted when I was going to get hungry, and I started cooking before I was chewing on the refrigerator's insulation strips for sustenance.

I had a plan for exercise too.

I think my mother bought the treadmill partly so I'd stop hating my father. A couple of years earlier our old treadmill had started making loud, rattling noises whenever I walked on it, like a huge cell phone set to vibrate. My dad then hauled it to an exercise equipment store to be repaired. When he was quoted the price for repairs, he left it at the store for scrap. I was devastated, because I saw the treadmill as my best hope for weight loss. I didn't have a job, so I couldn't pay for the repairs myself. I was a hamster without a wheel to run in—a very fat hamster.

Even though money was tight after my dad left, Mom celebrated the new year by spending several hundred dollars on a treadmill. She was worried about my health and knew I'd kept up with walking indoors in the past. She couldn't click an "undo" button for Dad's actions, but she could fix this one mistake.

Then the treadmill sat in our spare room for a year.

When it was first delivered, I walked on it four days in a row, inhaling that new-exercise-equipment smell as I strolled along. Then I redirected that use of electricity to the television set. Now, nearly a year after the delivery men had dropped off the heavy piece of machinery in my old bedroom, I laced up my tennis shoes and stepped on its foot panels once again. I slipped the magnetic key into the power console and clipped the end of the attached string to my waist. The key would automatically slide out and shut off the treadmill if I stumbled. I'd still fall on my face, but at least the tread wouldn't sand my eyebrows off. I hoped I could keep up with the breakneck speed of two and a half miles per hour.

I carefully adjusted the settings on the huge console as if I were plotting a complex trip through hyperspace. Then my cat crawled onto the tread. He flung his body down whimsically beneath me, lazing about as though my legs formed the apex of his throne. I could learn a lot about confidence from my kitty, who had never let his weight problem get in the way of his schemes to rule the world. But my need for exercise trumped any plans he had for megalomania.

The fastest way to get a cat off a treadmill is by hitting the start button.

The control panel emitted a few small beeps like a dump truck backing up, though I swear I didn't move an inch. As the pneumatics hissed to change the elevation, I started a slow and steady pace of two and a half miles per hour. This would be fast if I had legs the length of a Chihuahua's. At my weight it was all I could handle. I had a wide stance because of my thunder thighs, so I walked close to the edges of the tread. I lightly grasped the side rails during each step so I wouldn't fall off. My poor form might strain my muscles, but it made me feel safer. I huffed and puffed enough to demolish any little pigs' houses in the vicinity. I trundled forward until I was exhausted, gratefully pressing the big red STOP button and resting on the front rail as my motionless feet slid slowly behind me, leaning me forward like a ski jumper. I glanced at the flashing display.

Four-tenths of a mile. It was a start.

Eventually I started taking the stairs at work again, this time pausing on each floor to catch my breath and let people go by on the spacious landings. The stairwell itself was too narrow to let people zoom past me. I was like an overturned double-wide semi blocking the highway, preventing people from passing. When I reached my destination on the fourth floor, I stopped for a full minute at the top of the stairwell to catch my breath. I didn't want to walk down the hallway and into my office out of breath and red-faced. I was thankful that people who passed me avoided eye contact. I would do my best to ignore them too and pretend my face was red solely from exertion and not embarrassment.

I started parking farther out in parking lots. This worked exercise into my daily routine and also made it incredibly easy to find a parking spot. My former modus operandi when attacking a parking lot was to loop up and down the aisles like a needle passing back and forth through fabric until I found a spot near the door. In college, the lack of parking spots on campus led to particularly predatory habits. Frequently I would shadow people, humming the theme to *Jaws* quietly to myself until they reached their cars and evacuated their parking spots. Then I'd pounce, filling the space rapidly like air hissing into a vacuum. Now I would just go up an aisle until I found a space and take it, no matter how far it was from the door. The time it took to walk from the outer limits of the parking lot was far less than the time I had previously spent hunting for the best spot. I wasn't just getting cardio, I was saving hours of my life.

I spent those saved hours on the treadmill, walking several nights a week after I came home from work. I had to keep walking even when I felt as if I'd left my lungs half a mile behind me. I had to keep moving my feet up the incline even when the muscle fibers in my thighs seemed flammable. Exercise became the process of building up a tolerance for pain. If I kept at this long enough, I would be able to trade my mattress for a bed of nails without caring.

It was surprising how much time this was taking. I had known it would take at least two years to reach my goal, but I didn't realize I'd be dedicating an hour or two every day to making meals and exercising. This was going to wreak havoc on my TV-watching schedule.

As with the cooking, I eventually didn't mind exercise, even if I didn't exactly love it. Walking became easier over the months. This was good because I was becoming more fit, and I enjoyed walking from the car to the front door of my office building without gasping, but it was annoying because I had to keep pushing myself harder, walking farther or faster, trying to find the point where I was exerting myself without risking injury. One sprained ankle and I'd have to stop walking to heal. Who knew if I'd be able to get back into the routine again? My habits were new and tremulous, delicately balanced on the tip of a fulcrum like a teeter-totter. Only the slightest push could tip everything out of equilibrium and send my butt crashing to the ground.

After the first week of walking, I was down four pounds. I explored the grocery store the next week and lost six more. The week after that, I was down another ten. Twenty pounds in three weeks. This was awesome! And kind of scary. It was considered healthy to lose only one or two pounds a week. I hoped I wasn't on a tapeworm diet after all.

If I didn't own the scale I wouldn't have known I'd lost weight. Twenty pounds out of 372 was only 5 percent of my body weight. There was a reason I had never noticed when I was gaining or losing weight.

It was like peeling rubber bands off a rubber-band ball, each band reducing the mass almost imperceptibly.

Even if I had kept up this insane pace, which probably would have induced kidney failure or death, it would have taken me ten months to reach my goal. My birthday was in the tenth month of the year, so I would definitely be a year older by the time I was thin. Ten months—I could create a whole other human being in that time and still have an extra month to decorate the nursery. I consoled myself by thinking that a year from now I'd be a year older anyway; I couldn't stop it from passing, but I got to decide what I did with that time.

About a month after I'd cracked open my cookbooks and wiped the cat hair off the treadmill, I was driving down the highway home from work, thinking about what I would make for dinner. The Parmesan chicken recipe had been tasty and pretty easy, but I'd set ground turkey out to thaw, so I should probably make something with that. As I sailed past the entrance to the movie theater filled with buttered popcorn, I had a sudden revelation. I would be doing this for the rest of my life. No more stopping at White Castle for handy little burgers I could hold in one hand and devour as I drove home. No more laps around the McDonald's drive-through. No more stopping at Dairy Queen, even though I had a coupon for a free Blizzard. Things had changed. Forever. I had started the long process of brainwashing myself into healthier habits. As the movie theater moved into my rearview mirror, I was overwhelmed with the idea that I'd be managing these habits for the rest of my life. I was going to live another ten to twenty years because of all this healthy eating too, so I'd be stuck doing it even longer.

This wasn't a "diet," it was a "lifestyle change." I didn't even know what the word "diet" meant anymore. Being on a diet implies that you eventually will go off the diet. I had decided not to do anything that I was not prepared to do for the rest of my life. I didn't want to plug a hole in the dam with my finger; I wanted to seal it with epoxy or concrete. "Don't get crazy," became my number one rule. When I was hungry, I ate. If I really, really, really wanted a food, I ate it. I didn't want to fixate on something I couldn't have only to binge on it later. I didn't count calories because I knew it would drive me insane, obsessing over every detail, although I did measure out reasonable portions for my meals. But I did tell my family that I was on a diet. It was simpler than saying, "I have changed my lifestyle," and sounded a lot less pompous. I *was* regulating my diet of food for the day, but I would never be able to stop without gaining back the weight. I wanted to lose the weight only once. I didn't want to be a dieting Sisyphus, burning calories rolling a gigantic donut up a hill only to eat it at the top, repeating the task eternally.

Two weeks after I changed my eating habits and actually developed some exercise habits, I was no longer tired in the afternoons. I didn't find myself dropping quarters in the vending machine for a three o'clock sugar fix. My menstrual cramps were significantly less painful. My hair was less oily. I was less moody, and I stopped snapping at my family. I fell asleep quickly and slept the night through.

I was also kind of horny.[1] Fat cells don't just sit around being fat; they also raise the level of a hormone called SHBG (sex hormone-binding globulin), which binds to testosterone and diminishes sex drive. By losing weight I was freeing up testosterone, which stimulated my libido.

All it took for me to feel better was to eat better and walk a little. For years I'd been a hypochondriac, wondering if every headache were a symptom of brain cancer. I'd enjoyed the temporary pleasure of ice cream and candies at the expense of feeling good all the time.

All this healthy living was starting to make me feel alive. I'd never even realized I felt half dead.

CHAPTER 6

Stumbling Blocks

There were a dozen yellow and red roses on my desk. There was no card, but I knew they were from my mom. They appeared in the middle of March after I'd lost forty pounds in two months to weigh 330 pounds. The flowers were a much better show of support than the Hershey's Kisses she'd given me on Valentine's Day. I didn't eat roses.

By the beginning of April, I was down another ten pounds. Bizarrely, I even lost seven pounds the week I ate too many Cadbury Creme eggs for Easter. I'd now lost the equivalent of the two tubs of kitty litter that I always struggled to carry inside from the car. I just had to repeat that loss three more times, but it wasn't going to happen on the same brisk schedule. For the next several months my rate of loss stabilized to about ten pounds a month. The rational part of my mind that worried about loose skin was glad that the rapid rate was decreasing, but the pleasure-seeking part of my brain was going to miss those thrilling months in which I lost five or six pounds a week. I'd been waiting my whole life to be thin. I didn't want to wait any longer.

Four months was the longest I'd ever been able to sustain a period of weight loss. My good mojo was partly my own doing and partly luck.

I was more educated than I'd ever been before. (I could name four types of fats, three macronutrients, and two types of cholesterol.) My plan focused on foods I could eat, which was a more positive approach than focusing only on foods I couldn't eat. I wasn't tempted by sour cream and onion potato chips because my family kept them out of the house or at least hidden under their beds. There were no stressful events to send me running to the frozen desserts section of the grocery store. My treadmill was still working, and we had a service plan this time in case it did break. I also knew that it would take more than a year to get to goal, so I was settling in for a long ride. There was no shortcut.

I was pretty sure my clothes were getting looser. All my pants had elastic waistbands, so I wasn't sure. My brother and mother claimed my face looked more slender, but they knew I'd been trying to become thinner. My boss and coworkers hadn't said a thing.

There was a box at the bottom of my closet marked SKINNY CLOTHES, which was full of garments that most people would have labeled FAT CLOTHES. My younger brother's girlfriend had seen the box one day and commented, "Huh, I have a box like that too." She wasn't even fat. Maybe every girl, fat or thin, has a box of skinny clothes in the closet, a box of hope waiting to be opened before its contents have gone out of style.

I pulled on a couple of the shirts. They fit. I pulled on a pair of pants and was able to walk around in them, but I'd have to wait another ten pounds if I wanted to sit down and breathe at the same time. I'd never cared much about clothes and had been perplexed by my friends who read lots of fashion magazines, but when I looked in the mirror, I felt so sexy and cool, at least in relation to how unsexy and uncool I'd felt just three months earlier. There might be something to this whole fashion thing after all.

Then I gained weight.

It was only two pounds, but it was the first time the numbers had gone up since I'd started monitoring my weight. My first instinct was to blame it on my menstrual cycle. I always lost less weight the week of my period. Then I'd lose several pounds the week afterward. My body was retaining water, so even though I hadn't gained fat I had gained weight. The scale was too stupid to notice this. I felt bad for all the women who competed on *The Biggest Loser* show, since they were obviously at a disadvantage compared to the men thanks to this fluke of the menstrual cycle.

My girly hormones might also explain why I'd felt the need to eat a Reese's Peanut Butter Cup from the vending machine that week. I hadn't been walking as much lately, either. I wasn't being completely lazy; I'd just had two colds in three weeks, and I already wheezed enough when I exercised. If I tried breathing through a layer of phlegm, I might suffocate. I spent evenings on the couch instead, worrying and fretting that a microscopic virus might mark the end of my successful loss and herald the beginning of a long gain. Small slides were how bad habits started. A few days off could become a few weeks, and then a few months, until I was left wondering where it all went wrong. I needed to get back into the routine before the path I'd worn down was overgrown with weeds.

Of course, the cold might make me lose weight. The chicken broth diet was probably slimming.

I was also starting to get bored. Bored with my food. Bored with walking. Weight loss was a repetitive task. Eat right, exercise, sleep, repeat. Forever. I opened up my cookbooks again and looked for new recipes that wouldn't require me to buy something weird like muskrat root. I had to keep answering the same question every night, "What are you having for dinner?" I was sick of it. Why couldn't other people answer the question for me? And then do all the cooking? And while they were at it, could they lose all this weight for me too? My family had erratic work hours and could not be counted on to cook dinner regularly, so I was responsible for all of my own meals. The year before I would have just gone to McDonald's or Taco Bell if I didn't want to prepare something. Now that wasn't an option. Instead, I was leaving plates of leftover food in the microwave for my shocked yet grateful mother.

I noticed I wasn't sweating during my walk as much as I used to, so I kicked up the treadmill speed by a couple of tenths of a mile and increased the incline. I didn't enjoy hauling my huge ass up the slight hill, but I did it anyway.

I was doing a lot of things I didn't particularly want to do. I suppose that might be the definition of discipline. I had to override my desire to do what I wanted in the short term to get what I wanted in the long term. I couldn't support the fast-food industry and expect to get a slender body. Living healthy took so much time and effort. I'd barely worked on my other personal projects since I'd started. My bag of crochet work looked so lonely leaning against the bookcase, but I doubted needle arts burned many calories.

There was a battle raging between two parts of myself, Current Me and Future Me. Current Me was gung-ho about losing weight, eating healthy, and eschewing the elevator in favor of the stairs. Future Me would think about how close the convenience store was and how easy it would be to buy a bag of Reese's Pieces without anyone's knowing. I hated that bitch. Those two girls were locked in an endless boxing match with an infinite set of rounds.

Then one day Future Me bought a pint of Ben & Jerry's ice cream.

I had made a few small transgressions from my eating plan out of ignorance. I'd bought a salad at a fast-food place and later looked up the nutritional information online, only to discover the dressing had more fat than I did. The server went rather heavy on the bacon bits too, as if he were flinging pork confetti at a parade. If we were playing the blame game, I didn't deserve a penalty for that. I did deserve a foul for the ice cream.

I collapsed on the couch after work, sick of writing code and sick of the headache that Excedrin had not cured. I was out of Lean Cuisines and yogurt and diet sodas, and I knew I had to go to the grocery store if I wanted to eat lunch tomorrow. I looked at my reflection in the TV set, trying to talk my likeness into going to the store for me. She just sat on the couch and stared back at me.

There was *one* good reason to go to the store. That's where they kept the ice cream. I suddenly wanted to get off the couch. I returned with lots of healthy food and one pint of ice cream. A half hour later only the healthy food was left.

I felt so much better. I hadn't had any ice cream since December. Strangely, I didn't even feel all that bad about eating it. I hadn't purposely strayed from my diet since I'd started. It felt good to break the perfect spree. In high school I'd gotten all As for three years. By senior year I wasn't just scared of bees with wings and stingers but of big ones in capital letters on my report card. I'd been academically perfect for so long that it would have been traumatic to screw up right before becoming valedictorian. I managed to sustain my streak through high school, but when I got a B in my first semester of college, I was relieved. Being perfect was way too exhausting. I'd had my ice cream. I'd enjoyed it. My perfect dieting streak was broken. Now I'd just get back on track and make sure this didn't become a habit.

I lost a pound that week anyway. I hadn't even walked for three days. My body made absolutely no sense. Some weeks the scale was a distracted referee who missed reprimanding me on a foul. Other weeks it made a bad call despite my lack of errors.

I didn't feel bad about chomping down on the cherry chocolate chip ice cream, but I did determine its caloric content: 1,040 calories.

That was not something I'd done before. In my previous life, I'd gone back for two or three soft-serve ice cream cones at the all-you-can-eat Sizzler buffet and never regretted it at all. Now I had a heightened awareness of how different foods would affect my body, and I doubted I could ever flip off the light switch on this enlightenment. I'd always vaguely known that a Double Quarter Pounder with Cheese was bad for me, but discovering it had 740 calories was shocking. That was half a day's worth of food for some people. Fleshing out the details was like the difference between knowing there was a war going on in another country and seeing photos of a child mutilated by a land mine. The specific was far more shocking than the generalization.

It didn't seem to hurt me that badly anyway. Only a couple of weeks later, at the beginning of June, I stepped on the scale and a smile curled on my face when I saw the number 298. I was out of the 300s! I could weigh myself on regular bathroom scales now! I realized this milestone was just a fluke of our base-ten numbering system. If we had eight fingers I probably would have gotten excited when I hit 320 pounds, which is 500 in octet. But I wasn't going to let mathematical overanalysis get in the way of a party. I was under 300 pounds! I was already one-third of the way to my goal after only four and a half months. There was no reason to feel bad about canoodling with Ben & Jerry from time to time.

The next time I ate ice cream I felt differently.

The woman backing out of the parking spot behind me at the bookstore had not mastered the ability to drive and talk on her cell phone at the same time. The price of my brother's birthday gift card was twenty bucks, but it cost me $700 damage to my back driver's side door. I came home and ate his cupcakes. And some ice cream. And some cake the next day. And then some cookies for the Fourth of July, though by that point I'd already been awarded a check by the driver's insurance company, so I had no good excuse for pigging out. I'd actually earned money from the accident. At best I could claim that I thought the sounds of fireworks were signs of the coming Apocalypse and I'd decided to go out with my mouth mashed full of snickerdoodles. Two weeks later I was so tired of cooking dinner that I decided to buy an Extra Value Meal at McDonald's.

"No! Don't do it!" my brother called from the kitchen as I escaped through the back door. I pretended I didn't hear him. My family's support had gotten me a long way, but it wasn't going to get me to the drive-through.

My first ice cream indulgence had been an isolated incident, but this was becoming a multiple-week bender. I felt bad, not just emotionally, but physically. All that sugar made me sleepy and moody. I'd forgotten how much better I felt when I ate well. I'd gone through most of my life in a sugar coma and I had no desire to go back. I didn't want to become someone who apologized whenever she ate a piece of cake, but I couldn't recklessly eat whatever I wanted to anymore, either. If I did that I'd be trading my fortieth birthday cake for a daily injection of insulin.

Thankfully there were no birthdays to celebrate for several months. By now my healthier ways had become habits that I was able to pick up again. I'd never dropped them completely anyway, just fumbled the ball a couple of times without letting it completely hit the ground. Besides, I didn't have much else to do. I hadn't made many friends since we'd moved out of state several years ago. Friday nights were not spent at clubs with techno music blasting through speakers; they were spent on the treadmill with techno music blasting through my tinny earphones.

I still resented the fact that I had to bother with any of this. I'd never dieted because I wanted eating to be simple. This was complicated. I felt ridiculous counting out exactly thirty pistachios for my midafternoon snack. If I counted out twenty-nine by mistake, was

I going to be chewing on the plastic bag in ravenous hunger before lunch? If I counted out thirty-one was I doomed to a life of obesity? I wished I could instinctively eat whatever I wanted without worrying, but the last time I'd done that I'd gained 200 pounds.

I was still confused about what was "good" or "bad" for me. A dozen cookies were definitely bad, but one cookie was okay, right? When did the number of cookies I ate become too high to be part of a healthy diet? I didn't know, so I stuck to a small set of foods that I knew were "safe." I was hesitant to try anything new that might screw me up. I was still wrapping my head around all the new information I'd learned in the past five months. My brain was full. I wanted to find a place where I was nutritionally responsible but still indulged occasionally without giving myself unnecessary reprimands. A life without ice cream wasn't a life worth living.

But I still had to live in a world that made healthy eating as easy as stuffing my ass into size 4 jeans. I'd avidly avoided eating out with friends or relatives while I was relearning how to eat. Reprogramming my brain was hard enough without having to deal with the social pressures of eating. Picking the healthiest item on a menu was going to be my advanced dieting entrance exam. I managed to put it off until the beginning of August, when I'd lost ninety pounds and weighed 282 pounds. My mom had a steak house gift card, which we decided to use to celebrate the fact that the day ended in a "y." I fearfully stared down a menu full of deep-fried items. I searched through the menu, looking for the one item that wasn't covered in butter or soaked in saturated fats.

"What is the chicken fried in?" I asked the waitress.

"Lard," she replied. Damn, the restaurant wasn't even bothering to lie about it. I'd seen buckets of lard sold at the grocery store and wondered why it didn't sell 45-millimeter handguns next to them so you could just shoot yourself in the "baking needs" aisle.

The waitress started to place a basket of bread on the table. I looked at my mother tensely. I didn't want to fill up on empty calories, but I didn't want to stop her from enjoying some hot rolls if she wanted them.

"I don't really need any bread, but if you want to..." I trailed off, shrugging.

"No bread for us," she told the waitress. "My daughter's lost a lot of weight," she said proudly. I looked down at my menu, somewhat embarrassed but hiding a small smile behind the laminated paper. I got the impression my mother wanted me to tell our server how much weight I'd lost, but I didn't like to say unless directly asked. I didn't want to brag, especially considering the fact that I was still very obese. If I said I'd lost ninety pounds I bet most people would have thought, *Damn, you must have been* humongous *before.*

I was tempted by the "bad" foods on the menu. I knew it was hypothetically possible to eat fried foods and potato salads in small portions and still lose weight, but that style of eating was beyond me. I didn't want to screw up what seemed to be working with a plate of french fries.

I skipped over the fried mushrooms in favor of the steamed vegetables, though I honestly would have preferred the fried mushrooms. The word "lard" kept echoing in my head, which made the decision easier. I talked to my lunch companion instead of stuffing my face with bread while waiting for the main meal. I ordered water instead of a soda. It was strange behavior. Wearing the menu on my head as a hat would have appeared normal in comparison.

The strangest thing was that I could now slide into the booth without my belly brushing against the table. I even had three inches to spare. It was the small things in life that mattered, and I was definitely getting smaller.

CHAPTER 7

The Incredible Shrinking Woman

"**H**ey lady, have you lost weight?"

Saundra, the artist who worked down the hallway from me, was calling me "lady" because she couldn't remember my name, but I didn't care because she was the first person who did not share some of my DNA to comment on my weight loss. I had to lose only the equivalent of a small antelope to hear it.

"Oh yeah, I have," I said, not quite sure how to react.

"You look great!" she said with a chipper smile. She seemed genuinely happy for me.

"Oh, uh, thanks," I said as a grin crossed my face of its own volition, as if my mouth muscles had declared a coup against my visage. She was complimenting me. I knew there was a graceful way to take a compliment, but I hadn't yet learned what that was. I'd have to Google that when I got back to the office.

I wasn't used to being the center of attention. It's possible I gained weight so I wouldn't have to be. But if I were going to get thinner, I was going to have to deal with the fact that other people were going to notice. I'd been noticing it myself.

Lately, I had liked to play "Is she fatter than me?" It was a game that could be played anywhere, in the produce aisle of the grocery store, in line at the pharmacy, or even in the comfort of your own home as you watched television. All it required was a working pair of eyes and another female in your line of sight. You compared the size and shape of your body to that of your competitor's until you determined who was fatter. The thinnest girl won. The prize was a mix of smug satisfaction and self-disgust that you were playing the game at all.

I never used to play this sport because I always lost. I was fatter than everyone. It was a zero-sum game, but now I could win occasionally. I liked winning, but I also felt that it made me a very bad person. I shouldn't have to feel good about myself by putting down someone else. Certainly it shouldn't have been another female who struggled in the same culture as I did, which put such great value on what a woman looks like. We should be helping each other out, not cutting each other down.

Yet I constantly sized people up, male or female, fat or thin, so I knew what my relationship in society was to them. Was this person prettier than me? Was this person smarter than me? Did she have more money? Did he have more power? I needed to know where I stood in relation to others so I knew how to act around them. Frequently that first impression was determined by looks.

It was particularly silly because at 275 pounds I still had more than 100 pounds to lose. I was so much thinner, but people who passed me on the street knew nothing about my metamorphosis. They still categorized me as a fat girl when they did their own internal audit of my looks. The women I was now thinner than could have lost weight too. How would I know? Yet I still enjoyed seeing women who were fatter than me. I liked to remember where I came from.

My body had changed so much since then. I could fit my ass in a seat at the movie theater without my hip fat piling up against the cup holder. After I lost another six pounds to weigh 269, I was no longer morbidly obese, according to my BMI. It was just vanilla-flavored obesity for me. I was finally at a point where the weight-loss ads on TV would sometimes list my current size as someone's "before" weight. I was probably the only 269-pound woman in the world who felt skinny, but compared to my old self I was a willow.

I felt a twisted sense of satisfaction that I had more weight to lose than anyone I knew, as though this would make my final accomplishment all the more grand. In school I would sometimes trade eyeglasses with a classmate and whoever had the worst vision "won," as if you'd confirmed you had more of a right to four eyes than the other person. I felt the same odd superiority knowing that I might one day be able to say I'd lost 210 pounds, as if weight loss were a competition.

I felt like a winner as my body changed. When I was driving to work later that week I asked the windshield, "Has that building been painted?" The windshield never answered me, but I was pretty sure the siding hadn't been that white the day before. I didn't know what color the building had been previously, but I knew it had changed. That's how I felt about my body.

While lying in bed one night, I rolled on my side and adjusted my legs on top of one another so my knees were touching. I suddenly noticed I could feel bones beneath the skin where previously there had been a cushy layer of fat. It was as if someone had popped the Bubble Wrap around my legs. I rubbed my hand up my side and could feel the outline of my pelvic bone. My gynecologist had told me I had a pelvis, but I thought she was just starting a rumor. Was it possible I might have a skeletal system too? I'd seen my foot bones in an x-ray when I banged my toe on the stairwell as a child, but I sometimes doubted my other bones existed because they were tucked tightly under a comforter of fat.

I didn't have any distinct memories of what my knees or my hips felt like one hundred pounds earlier, but they *seemed* different. When I continued feeling up my side like a clumsy high school boy, I could feel my ribs and count how many I had. One, two, three, four, not as chubby as before. The next day when I rubbed my chin in thought, I noticed I was trying to roll the skin farther than was possible. My body was melting like an iceberg. I might be discovering a frozen caveman between my butt cheeks soon.

For months, whenever I put my hands on my hips and felt the edge of a bone I also felt a split second of surprise. Previously I had thought it was uncomfortable to rest my hands in fists on my hips like Peter Pan, but I realized it wasn't that hard when you could actually settle them into the curve of the bone. It wasn't much longer before my collarbones started to emerge. I tapped on them like a xylophone while staring at the computer screen.

My body was finally catching up with the way my mind had always perceived it to be. Anorexics have body dysmorphic disorder, which makes them think they are fatter than they actually are. Even when their ribs show through their flesh, in their heads they think they're fat. Mentally I seemed to have an inverted form of anorexia, unable to truly grasp how fat I was.

The image of myself in my head was that of normal weight. If I were to draw a picture of myself, I'd make myself skinnier than I was without really noticing. In the movie *The Matrix,* this illusion was called residual self-image. Even though the character of Neo had a closely shaved head of hair in the real world, he had a full head of hair in the cyber reality of the Matrix. I was fat, I knew I was fat, yet if I were to enter the Matrix, I would have been thin.

This was clear if you looked at any of my Internet avatars, the icons I used on message boards or instant messenger to represent myself. Online everyone can exist in soft lighting, with Vaseline smeared on the camera lens. I sent the prettiest, most lovely version of myself out there, online or off. Unfortunately I couldn't digitally erase the zit on my cheek before a date.

The desire to look good was evident in my "fat girl angle shot." Classic signs: looking up at the camera to hide a double chin, high contrast, cropped from the neck up. My first online photo was a textbook example, complete with a high camera angle, hair across my face, and cavelike lighting—all obvious attempts to hide my fatness, or the fact that I could barely afford light bulbs.

This mental image was shaken whenever I saw photos of myself looming large over a thinner person standing next to me. One night I forgot to pull the venetian blinds down on the window next to my computer desk and was completely disgusted when I caught the eye of my reflection in the window. As I sat at my desk, the fat puddled all around me, particularly in my thighs and belly, making me look larger than I'd ever imagined possible. I quickly pulled the curtains closed.

The living color of video made me curse the invention of the cathode-ray tube. In my college speech class, all our speeches were taped. We had to review our performances to critique ourselves after each speech. The round, obese girl on the video was out of sync with the image of myself in my head. I did not move like that. I did not look like that. I could watch only a couple of seconds at a time, and then I'd fast-forward through the freak show, my sped-up swaying making me look like a bowling pin about to topple. When I was done, I took care to tape over my five minutes of arguments about why Indiana should adopt daylight saving time, erasing the image from existence in a way I'd never been able to do in real life.

Even though I could see the difference in the mirror or on a tape, these moments of clarity lasted less than a minute. For the majority of my day, I did not look at myself. I looked at other people. I was like a dog raised by cats who thinks she's a kitten. It seemed to me that most people in the world were only mildly overweight or of average size. When I'd been my fattest, finding someone who was as obese as me was rare. Being surrounded by people who weren't enormous made me think that I looked like them too.

Even when I worked with other fat people, I dissociated myself from them. At one job, I worked with an overweight, diabetic middle-aged woman. She would trudge slowly from the door to her chair like the air was made of thick chocolate syrup that she struggled to plow through. On some level, I knew that I could be her in twenty years, yet I would separate myself from her in my mind. She was not like me. I was not *that* fat. I did not look like that, though most likely I did. And even if I did, I still had time to avoid that fate if I got my ass off my ergonomic chair.

This erroneous self-image is partly what prevented me from acknowledging my weight problem. Even as the pounds kept piling on, my self-image remained skinny and allowed me to live comfortably in denial of the problem creeping up around me.

I hadn't successfully eliminated all video imagery of my fat years, though. I was sorting through old data CDs and files on my computer when I found a video I shot for film class in college. It starred my cat, Officer Krupke, and revealed what he did when I left my apartment. It started to the bouncy tones of "What's New, Pussycat?" but as soon as I left my place, "Cat Scratch Fever" kicked in and Krupke proceeded to order catnip online, watch Catwoman on TV, raid the fridge, and place his butt on my scanner for a cat scan. I was pleased to find that it was funny, but what wasn't funny was how huge I was.

Had I really been that large and lumbering? I seemed to waddle like an overgrown penguin. I'd destroyed all my speech class videos, but I had forgotten about this piece of footage. Seeing pictures of my old, morbidly obese self was jarring, but seeing how all that weight had made me move was shocking.

I caught a shot of my refrigerator on the video as Krupke stole some sliced turkey from the second shelf. My eyes raised in judgment when I saw twenty-four-packs of regular, nondiet soda on the shelves. I wasted hundreds of calories a day sipping that liquid candy, making me fatter without filling me up.

My younger brother Jim had played the catnip delivery man, so I dragged him over to my computer to share in the shock. His jaw hit the keyboard hard enough to type nonsense words and leave keyboard marks on his chin. I was fat. He was fat. We were both so fat!

Could people really comprehend their own physical changes without the proof of photographs and videos? Now you can buy a disposable camera at any drugstore, but affordable cameras have been available to most people only within the past century. Some people could have had drawings made or portraits painted, but that was probably beyond the budget of the average person. Even if you did sit for a painting, how much of the difference in your looks would you attribute to actual change, and how much to the artist's interpretation?

Without my fat pictures and videos, I might not have believed how much I'd physically transformed. After those speedy first months the weight had come off slowly, just like it had arrived, slithering in and out of my life. There were days when I prayed I could wake up thin. I'd wish that I could raise a magic sword above my head, yell some enchanted words, and undergo a transformation sequence complete with glitter and sparkles and an unseen chorus singing my theme song, transforming me instantly from fat to thin. But if my shock at seeing my old fat self was any indication, perhaps it was better that I was transforming slowly. If I were to suddenly wake up in a thin body, I wouldn't know how to act. It's easy to say, "Just be yourself," but who I was had been shaped by how other people treated me, and right or wrong, that was determined by how I looked.

As strange as this transformation was for me, I was not entirely sure how it affected other people in my life. My boss hadn't mentioned the subject. He'd complained that staring at a computer monitor all day for the last decade had hurt his vision, but if he hadn't noticed that I was no longer in danger of breaking our cheap office chairs, he should have been checked for cataracts. My boss was friendly and easygoing, so I thought he would at least mention my metamorphosis in passing after the first hundred pounds, but day after day I sat in my office chair without a word from him about my appearance. At least if I one day transformed into a gigantic beetle I wouldn't have to worry about my job security, provided I learned to type with my antennae. It wasn't until I was weighing in under 200 pounds and told him I was writing a book about my weight loss that I first broached the topic. He said he had definitely noticed and had wanted to compliment me, but he was just playing it safe since he didn't know how to tactfully approach the subject. It can be difficult to compliment someone's weight loss without implying she looked like a big, fat blob before. As a man and as my boss, he was also hesitant to say anything about my appearance for fear that it would be misinterpreted as flirtation or harassment.

The dynamic between female friends could be tricky too. My oldest friend, Cristy, hadn't been returning my phone calls. We met when we were both thin second-graders, and then we both got fat. I had gained weight first and felt a twisted sort of happiness a couple of years later when she started gaining too. I liked that I wasn't alone in the elastic waistband. A year earlier I had Photoshopped a picture of us so we both looked thinner. I was moving that image into the real world, but the supermodel-thin version of my friend still existed only in the picture frame. Cristy lived several hours away, so I saw her only a couple times a year. She'd never been in contention for the title of "World's Best Email Correspondent," nor had she been good at that old thing we used to do with envelopes and paper and pens, either.

It wasn't uncommon for us to go months without talking to each other, but the silence was starting to become extreme. We had talked on the phone a couple of times, and I'd told her I had lost a lot of weight. I'd gotten some emails since then and a postcard from a Disney cruise, but that was it. The first ten months I attributed this to Cristy's being her regular, busy, communication-challenged self. She was married, worked a full-time job, and went to school part time. As I flipped more pages on my monthly calendar, I got the creeping suspicion that my weight loss might be pushing us apart. How had my decrease in size made her feel? I thought she was genuinely happy for me, but that joy might be laced with pain. I wanted to lose weight, not friends. If the situation were reversed, I'd probably be jealous of her for doing something I couldn't. I hoped that wouldn't stop me from returning her calls. I was the same person, just in different packaging. She might be unsure that the stuff inside was still the same, as I had been when the manufacturer had changed the design of my favorite yogurt cups.

I hoped I was being paranoid and Cristy was just being Cristy. There might be something else going on with her that had nothing to do with me or with the continental drift in the tectonics of our relationship. The longer this went on, the more shocking it would be when we eventually did see each other again. What if it got to the point where she walked past me without recognizing me? If I dyed my hair, got contact lenses and a nose ring, I'd be more incognito than a member of the Witness

Protection Program. I called her sometimes, but I usually got voice mail because she worked a third-shift job and I worked nine to five.

After sixteen months, I finally met up with Cristy at a women's study conference close to my city. I had lost about 150 pounds since I'd seen her last. I was in the back of the room when she hurried in to present her project. I snuck up behind her, braced for her unpredictable reaction. She smiled and exclaimed, "Jennette!" and got up to embrace me in a hug, fitting her arms around my entire body for once. "You look great!" she said with a smile in her eyes and not just on her mouth.

I was relieved she recognized me. We spent the rest of the day together and I purposely avoided talking about anything related to weight. I had always wondered why no one had staged an intervention on me when I was almost 400 pounds. I got my answer when I was far too chicken to ask one of my best friends if she hated me because I was thinner. It would have been impossible to do without bringing up the topic of her own weight, and I really didn't want to go there. I even made a point of eating the chocolate fudge brownie served with lunch just to show that I wasn't a dieting Nazi who wanted everyone to eat tomato salads. If I had still been fat, I might have avoided eating the chocolate dessert just to show everyone that fat people didn't subsist only on brownies. Both approaches were rather dumb. I doubt that anyone cared what I ate for lunch. I don't remember what anyone else had. My lunch was not a political statement.

It wasn't until I was weighing in under 200 pounds and told her I was writing a book about my weight loss that I brought up the topic. The secret to approaching your friends and coworkers about an uncomfortable topic: Write a book about it. It just becomes research. As she put it, "I was thrilled for you and super jealous. And while I wasn't overtly avoiding you (I just suck), I know it crossed my mind as to how this would change our friendship, both in good and 'bad' ways.

Like getting ice cream together, or something. I love you, and I'm both ecstatic and awed by your hard work and great results. Whatever issues I have with my fat ass have nothing to do with our friendship, except that now you're my role model, too."

We still go out for ice cream together.

CHAPTER 8

The Girl in the Mirror

The restroom mirror was missing.

This was a problem because I could not check out how cute I was. I used to wish there were no mirrors in the world, like the king and queen's campaign to have all the spinning wheels destroyed in Sleeping Beauty's kingdom. But now I looked forward to going to the ladies' room during my work day so I could see how much skinnier I had become. I needed to confirm that fact every few hours. I was afraid the front paunch might reappear while I was typing.

It had been a year and I still wasn't thin. I weighed 242 pounds, down 130, but still obese according to my body mass index. I was feeling much skinnier. I actually weighed eight pounds less than what my driver's license said. If workers at the Department of Motor Vehicles had a dollar for every pound people have lied about on their driver's licenses, they wouldn't have to work at the DMV anymore. The last time I weighed this much, I felt so fat that I had speed walked past my reflection. Now I felt so thin that I was striking poses like I was in a Madonna video. If anyone wants to feel good about herself, gaining a hundred pounds and then losing it is one way to go. It made me feel like a superstar. Until the janitor hung a replacement mirror on the wall, my love affair with myself was going on a break. I'd have to wait until I could go home and admire myself between the toothpaste spittle spots on my own bathroom mirror.

I had never been vain before. I didn't know how to apply eyeliner without scraping my cornea. I shaved my legs as frequently as new Supreme Court justices were appointed. My lack of concern about my image probably helped me gain so much weight in the first place. Those days were over. The mirror let me admire the results of my hard work and recalibrate my self-image on a daily basis as I shrank.

There is a painting by Pablo Picasso called *Girl Before a Mirror* that depicts a woman in warm colors looking at her reflection in an oval-shaped, floor-length mirror. Her mirror twin is painted in cold colors with a slightly different appearance, as though the girl can't see herself as she really is, or the way the world sees her isn't the way she is inside. I'd had a print of this painting hanging in my living room for years, but I felt like I understood it more than I ever had before. I certainly felt beautiful, but I wasn't sure if what I saw in the mirror was the same thing people were seeing outside the looking glass. I didn't know if it even mattered.

I returned to my office desk and crossed my legs one over the other. I was crossing my legs all the time now just because I could. A year ago I was as likely to be able to cross my legs as I was to run cross-country. Now my thighs were slim enough to accommodate the proper angle required for this traditional ladylike pose. I looked at my wristwatch as I began to type and noticed I was down four notches on the band, about an inch. I was amazed there had been that much fat in my wrist; I thought the skin there covered only bone and veins and ligaments. My best excuse for not giving blood was rapidly disappearing. Nurses had always had trouble finding my veins, but now my arms sported faint blue lines scattered under my translucent skin instead of the red stretch marks I'd so hated. The scores of stretch marks on my belly had faded to a shiny color, like streaks of raindrops on a windshield. If I inhaled deeply they would pucker slightly out from my body. They were my fat scars.

I still had about eighty pounds to lose before I hit my arbitrarily determined goal weight. When I was washing all my flabby bits in the shower, I started to wonder exactly how that excess weight was distributed. It was like trying to guess the number of jelly beans in a jar. My belly alone must have had at least twenty-five pounds. I guessed at least another twenty-five pounds in my ass. If my arms had five pounds each, that would leave twenty pounds in my legs. That couldn't be right. Maybe my ass wasn't as big as I thought? Unfortunately, I couldn't swivel my head around to check because I wasn't possessed by the devil, I'd just have to go with what I saw in the mirror. I could have been overestimating my arm weight. The upper arms looked like bat wings, but how much did they really weigh? I was hesitant to underestimate them since I'd never suspected there could be so much fat in my wrist.

My mother insisted that my shoe size would get smaller too, but I didn't think I had that much fat in my feet. I had heard a snide comment or two about the size of my ass, but no one had ever accused me of having chunky toes. There wasn't a special shoe store for fat people. But she argued that my arches might become less bowed as my weight decreased, which could cause me to go down a size or two.

As I continued working, I felt chilly despite the sweater buttoned up over my long-sleeve shirt. I felt cold lately, and I was considering investing in a space heater. Either that or I'd break down my absent coworker's desk to build a fire on top of the photocopier. I could use my Lean Cuisine packaging for kindling. At first I had been convinced that my office was cold because it was situated in a converted warehouse that had self-washing floors. The fact that water leaked between the window frames during thunderstorms had to have been a new age design scheme, not a sign of rust and decay and poor insulation from the elements. My boss didn't think it was cold, but I had always suspected he was an alien from the planet of lava men.

To prove that I wasn't crazy, I bought an indoor-outdoor thermometer and took it into the office. Then I said some naughty words and stopped at the drugstore the next day to buy one AAA battery. I popped it into the thermometer and waited to see if my working conditions were horrible enough to warrant a lawsuit.

It was 72.6 degrees Fahrenheit.

I was wearing a lightweight sweater, a blazer, and a blouse, and I still felt as if I'd been locked in a freezer. I guessed my body was either missing the warm insulation of my fat or reacting to my weight loss by lowering my metabolism. There wasn't much I could do about it besides investing in wool socks.

I wasn't just looking better, I was feeling healthier too. When I later got down to 225 pounds, I stopped at the blood-pressure machine at the pharmacy. I stuck my hand through the cuff so it could be squeezed like a fresh melon. I was surprised that my arm fit somewhat comfortably and the machine didn't completely cut off my circulation when it choked my arm. The last time I'd used the machine I thought I'd have to gnaw my arm off at my elbow to exit the store. The cuff deflated and released my arm. I checked the numbers with anticipation as if I were hoping for a high score on Tetris. The display read: 122/71. Woo-hoo! I wanted to take a victory lap around the feminine hygiene aisle, throwing tampons in the air like confetti. My family had a history of hypertension, but that reading was perfectly normal. I was glad to break from family tradition.

I checked the clock on my computer and saw that it was after five o'clock. I gathered up my things to leave and said goodbye to my boss. As I walked down the hallway I started to think about what to make for dinner that night and what exercises I needed to do before I started cooking. I was now eating like a thin person and exercising like a thin person, but I was still fat. If I ended a smoking habit, as soon as I took the last puff of smoke I could say I had quit. But after I'd started acting like a thin person, it was still going to take a long time to quit being fat.

Some people might say I had a skinny girl inside just waiting to get out. I hated that expression. It made sense only if I'd swallowed a Lilliputian for lunch who was fighting her way back up my esophagus. It sounded like something to say if you wanted to escape the moral judgments that came along with being fat. I translated it to, "I'm not really a fat person. I'm just a skinny person in disguise! I'm not a glutton who is worthy of your scorn. I'm a virtuous, little girl who just happens to have a slow metabolism."

I didn't believe I could split my personality in half like that. Splitting occurred when you tried to break an idea into binary oppositions. Someone was good or bad. She was a fat person or a thin person. Splitting occurred when a concept was too emotionally complex for you to handle. The skinny girl and the fat girl weren't different girls. Neither one was necessarily good or bad. They were both just girls; same great taste, one with less fat. Their differing sizes didn't change my underlying personality. I was depleting fat cells, not brain cells. I could be a lot of things, thin and fat among them, but neither one was any more my "true" identity. I could be a mouthy bitch if someone provoked me, but when I met a cute guy I would frequently be rendered mute. I wasn't a thin girl who had been temporarily possessed by a fat person. My size was just a reflection of the environment I was currently living in. I was simply whoever I was today; size may vary.

People seemed more comfortable categorizing me as just one thing, like a one-dimensional character in a bad horror movie. They liked to cast me in that role according to how I looked, as if I could weave my personality into flesh and wear it over my skeleton like a dress. I could control the image I projected to some extent. I had a sassy flip in my curly hair and I enjoyed the irony of my pink argyle socks speckled with skulls and crossbones, but those clothes were still just a costume. No one could ever know exactly who I was just by looking at me. Even if my smaller-size ass highlighted by my boot-cut jeans was a more accurate reflection of who I considered myself to be, it was still just a costume I was wearing over my bones. Yet we all still seemed to be kids playing dress-up out of the costume box in the classroom corner.

These costumes affected how I lived my life, just as if I'd tried squeezing into a corset and found I couldn't breathe. When I wore my fat-girl body, people avoided looking at me. I became an extra in the background of a movie. Now that I had a thinner body, I was being cast as a supporting actor, if not the lead. As I walked down the hall at work, a tall man with brown hair made eye contact with me and said, "Good evening." I waved good night to him in return. That was odd. It was happening more and more often. People were making eye contact. They were saying hello even if I didn't know them. They were being friendly for no apparent reason. Was this normal?

It definitely wasn't normal that I started being friendly and outgoing in return. When I bought a pair of tights at a store, the cashier started to make small talk with me about how cute they were. I wondered if she'd have bothered to chat with the morbidly obese version of myself. Most checkout clerks I'd encountered seemed to be suffering from posttraumatic retail stress and hated all customers. Usually when I bumped into sales associates while shopping I would cower in fear when they asked the dreaded question, "Can I help you?" No matter how unenthusiastically they delivered the query, I didn't want their help. I wanted to get in and out with as little human contact as necessary. I'd usually mumble something and slink away. Now I found myself able to flash a perfect smile and say in a chipper voice, "No, thanks," before I resumed browsing.

When I went shopping for a used car, my mother and I went to a dealership where I waited for five minutes until a balding man finally sat down to help me. He began pushing me into a five-year loan at a high interest rate, trying to sell it as a deal even though I'd be paying more money than I had budgeted. I stayed firm and said I wasn't interested. As I got up to leave, he tried to get me to test-drive another car on the lot. I could smell the desperation on him. He mentioned that he'd just been transferred from the online sales department, and I wondered if his bosses were setting him up to fail and be fired. I felt sorry for him, but he didn't have anything I wanted to buy.

The salesman scrambled after me as I crossed the sidewalk to the car. I turned and said, "Thanks, but I'm just going to go now," in a polite and friendly tone. As I looked back at him I felt a surge of power that I'd rarely ever felt in my life. I was standing my ground, not bowing to the pressure another person was putting on me. It had been my habit to bend like a twist tie. I didn't know how to say no. It was such a simple syllable: No. I hadn't undergone speech therapy, but I was finding it easier and easier to say that short, simple word. I had lost a tremendous amount of weight. I had the power to change my world if I wanted to, and I didn't want my world to include an uncomfortable test-drive with a barely competent car salesman. I felt a high, despite the headache I'd developed from car-shopping dehydration. This was thrilling.

The fat girl hadn't done those things. She had flailed hopelessly for a forgotten line all alone on stage. The not-as-fat girl was being fed lines by her costars, who held out pieces of themselves that she could cling to. The world was more supportive now. In Picasso's painting, the girl stood alone with her reflection, but my reality was being shaped in many ways by other people. I was like the mirror, reflecting back their goodwill.

I was getting a new body, so did I need to get a new personality too? If you've got the dress, you need the shoes. None of my old clothes fit anymore. I'd sold my fat jeans on eBay, but my sense of style hadn't changed. I was still the same person. I was just starting to share myself with the world. The smiles and friendly glances were coaxing me to come out of my protective shell. The world seemed to resent my presence far less. It was sad I had to lose weight to get that. I was boiling off the fat cells until all that remained was my undiluted self, 100 percent pure.

I walked to the parking lot and drove home to change into my workout clothes. I took a jog on the treadmill. I had been walking regularly for more than a year now. I was learning more about nutrition and training all the time. I was living such a healthy life, but people who looked at my flabby body probably had no idea. At what point did an activity become part of my identity? How many lumpy sweaters did I have to knit before people started thinking of me as a knitter? How many CD mixes did I have to burn before friends thought of me as a girl with good taste in music? How long would I have to eat well and exercise before I was no longer pretending to be a healthy, thin person and was actually considered one by myself and others?

My mother finally decided to sell the house. I needed to find an apartment or get really friendly, really fast, with our home's new owners. I took my mom apartment hunting with me since she always remembered to ask sensible questions like, "Is water included in the rental fee?" while I only made insightful comments such as, "The carpet sure is soft." We got out of the car at the first complex, and I was halfway to the rental office before I noticed I was suddenly alone. I turned around to see my mom lagging two or three yards behind me. Then I realized the shocking truth. I had become that which I used to hate—a fast walker.

People always walked faster than me and it really pissed me off. Whenever I had walked with my older brother, he would zip past me effortlessly, frequently stopping at corners waiting for me to catch up. I blamed it on his long legs. This theory was disproved when I walked with a shorter coworker to her farewell lunch the year before. I felt as if I were running down the sidewalk just to match her casual pace. She slowed down as we neared a crosswalk, like the hare waiting for the tortoise to catch up. I was embarrassed that she was breaking her regular stride to accommodate my slowness.

My mother weighed a bit more than me and was thirty years older, so it wasn't as though I were outpacing a roadrunner on crack, but when we'd visited New York City two years earlier we had trundled past street vendors at the same pace. I'd lightened my load since then.

It was hard to think that anyone was changing as much as I was. When I checked my email and blogs online, there was a new journal post by a friend from high school, who had been to a bar the night before and run into another high school friend. I assumed I would take the prize for most changed at our high school reunion, but I think Daniel might beat me, now that he was going by the name of Danielle.

I had known Daniel fairly well, but I knew the back of his head better. I had been positioned directly behind him in the opening box formation of our marching band halftime show. Clean scalp, no lice. I was disappointed I hadn't run into him at the bar myself, though it probably would have taken several minutes before we recognized each other. I imagine our conversation would have gone like this:

"Hey, didn't you used to be really fat?" she would say as she batted her curled eyelashes.

"Hey, didn't you used to have a penis?" I would reply while sipping a Diet Pepsi.

I never knew Daniel was unhappy with his gender, but I was happy to hear about his decision, even if it made pronoun usage particularly tricky. We had more in common than I'd thought. I certainly had experienced disliking my external appearance. I was also discovering what it was like to undergo a dramatic physical change. Danielle would surely know what it was like to meet old friends and see their jaws drop open in shock. I wasn't the only one becoming more myself. It was nice to be reminded that there was more than one way to do that.

I had flipped through a community education course catalog recently, contemplating taking one of its fitness classes since I was still too cheap to join a gym. On my way to the blurbs about cardio kickboxing and aerobic belly dancing, I kept stopping to read course descriptions for glassblowing, woodworking, and blacksmithing. I could make my own dumbbells or cast finger cymbals for the belly-dancing class. I could learn to paint like a Dutch master. There were so many possibilities contained between the cheap newspaper pages of the booklet. So many things that I could do or be. I had started losing weight so I could find myself, whoever I was hidden beneath the padding that kept me safe from the sharp corners of the world. But as Danielle probably already knew, I didn't need to find myself; I needed to create myself instead.

CHAPTER 9

Too Small for My Britches

In April I needed to buy new spring clothes yet again, because last year's T-shirts were falling off my 225-pound frame. This was fun at first, buying cute new clothes and feeling pretty. I hadn't felt pretty that often in my life, not since I'd worn pink patent leather shoes as a little girl. When I could finally fit into jeans at Lane Bryant again, I held a mini fashion show for the mirror in our front hallway. I pretended the trampled carpeting was a Paris runway and the clumps of cat hair were limelights. I proudly showed off my newly purchased size 28 jeans to the spider hiding in the moulding cracks. I imagined him applauding with four pairs of legs.

Now my cute new clothes no longer fit. It wasn't fair. All my clothes had expiration dates, like milk gallons, only they weren't stamped on the labels. I felt particularly bad if I wore something only a couple of times before it became too big. It was such a waste of money. The most expensive thing I'd bought was a new winter coat, because I didn't want to drop more than a hundred dollars on a garment that wouldn't fit next year. The only one benefiting from this was my mom, who was walking around the house in my old clothes, enjoying my free service as her personal shopper.

I had started experimenting with sewing so I could alter some of my favorite clothes. This worked for a few size decreases, but after a certain point the cut and shape of a garment was too different for me to remake it in a smaller size. Tank tops were pretty easy; I could just take in the sides, but eventually the arm straps would slide off my shoulders because they were set too far apart. Then I'd have to send them to Goodwill, knowing that I was playing an evil trick on the size-24 consumer, who would be horrified when she couldn't fit into the blue tank top I'd sized down to an 18.

I had wanted to knit a sweater during the past winter. My problem, besides the fact that I couldn't knit, was that I didn't know how big to make the sweater. Not only was I losing weight, but I didn't know how fast I could knit. The faster I lost weight, the smaller I would need to make it. But the faster I knit, the bigger I should make it. It was a calculus problem. I started to have flashbacks—eleventh-grade math, Mrs. Stewart, a word problem involving a lighthouse and a woman walking a dog on the beach. It was all coming back to me except how to actually do any of the math. I decided to just buy a sweater.

But then spring came, and it was time to start shopping again. I wandered out of the plus-size clothing department into the misses' section on a lark. I grabbed an extra-large T-shirt and walked to the dressing room. I pulled it on over my head, looked in the mirror, and saw that the shirt was baggy. I nearly fainted and hit my head on the doorknob. All my perfect attendance T-shirts from middle school had been XL. I couldn't remember ever buying a smaller size. I returned to the sales floor, grabbed a size large and returned to the dressing room. It fit well, hugging all the right spots.

It completely blew my mind.

I could now shop in the "normal" stores. I'd been banished for most of my life to the special plus-size retailers and the women's sections of department stores stowed far away from the misses' section, as if cellulite were contagious. The clothes for fat girls were not like the clothes for "average" girls. You had to pay twice as much for a product that was only half as stylish. The extra fabric didn't cost that much.

Fat-girl clothes were lousy with sequins. I suspected in lieu of daycare that many full-figured clothing stores allowed employees' children to run around with a bedazzler, applying shiny plastic beads to every tank top or blouse in sight. Designers probably thought fat women wanted to distract onlookers with shiny objects so no one would notice we were fat. Soon they'd be adding bells and rattles for further distractions.

There were a couple retailers that catered just to the plus-size market, but my options were limited to whatever they decided to stock that season. The year peasant skirts were in I would have joined a nudist colony if I hadn't been ashamed to be seen naked. In some ways the lack of selection made shopping very easy. I'd go to Lane Bryant, pick out the least ugly clothes in the store, and go home. Not much thinking required.

A lot of fat girls liked to bitch about Lane Bryant's clothes, I among them, but I also knew it wasn't Lane Bryant's fault that I didn't love everything in its windows. No single store could possibly serve the needs of all fat people. If you made all thin people shop at The Gap, there'd be a lot of unsatisfied customers complaining about its khakis. I couldn't understand why there weren't more plus-size stores. My local news station made it seem as if we were a nation of headless fat people. We were supposedly the first generation that would have shorter lifespans than our parents because of increasing obesity rates.[1] Shouldn't the plus-size clothing industry be a boomtown, with a Casual Male XL popping up next to every Taco Bell?

A few new plus-size retailers had set up shop in the past decade, but not as many as you'd think. Lots of them did most of their business online and didn't have many retail outlets. Even if I did order something online, I'd have to buy several sizes to be sure I found something that fit my shape. I'd also have to pay extra shipping to send back the unwanted items. I'd resorted to buying slacks online only after I realized I no longer fit into the biggest size at Lane Bryant, a 28. I had stretched out my last pair in that size until they were a thirty-something. Then I wore out the inner thighs. I had my mother patch them because it was too depressing to hunt for another pair.

I'd stopped wearing jeans after high school because I couldn't find them in my size. I'd resorted to slacks made out of a spandex/polyester blend. I couldn't wear denim without being mistaken for a gold miner's tent. A girl in one of my college classes wore jeans that appeared to be big enough for me. I was tempted to ask her where she bought them, but I couldn't do it because it would bring attention to the fact that she was fat. It was okay if I called myself fat, but it was forbidden to use the f-word about another girl. Evil high school boys called women fat, not other fat girls. If she brought it up first, then it would be okay, but otherwise it would be a hostile assault on a neighboring country. I would occasionally look over my shoulder at her during the boring parts of a lecture, trying to think of ways to bring the topic up, but I never did find out the location of the fat-girl denim store.

I usually shopped alone because my thinner friends and I couldn't find clothes at the same stores. This segregation seemed unfair, but it was probably for the best. If I'd had to sort through the 3X selections while a teenybopper at the next rack moaned about how huge she felt in size 4 jeans, I probably would have beaten her to death with a wooden clothes hanger. I was glad that the saleswomen at plus-size stores were fat girls. They were probably just there for the employee discount, but at least I knew they had no right to judge me or act superior.

While I was grateful for stores like Lane Bryant that kept me from wearing the latest in garbage bag couture, shopping at the fat-girl store always reminded me of how different I was.

Until now.

Sure, my pear shape mandated that I still wear size-26 jeans, but I could buy shirts at the "normal" stores. I felt as if I'd moved up a level while playing *Grand Theft Auto*. I could now access a whole new section of the game, only without all the stealing and shooting and whoring, although that would certainly have made the shopping experience more interesting. I went to Old Navy just so I could say I'd bought something there. I started getting more and more into fashion now that I actually had options.

Before I lost a lot of weight, I thought fashion was somewhat ridiculous. I didn't understand why a guy in my high school English class asked to read a copy of *Seventeen* after a classmate was through with it. I was a girl and even I didn't read those magazines. (This boycott probably saved me several knockout blows to my self-esteem.) I didn't watch daytime television either, but my mother had *Oprah* on her TiVo season pass, so I would catch snippets of episodes while walking around the house. One day the show did makeovers that made women look twenty pounds thinner just by changing their clothes. I bought the book it was promoting the very next day.

When I started reading about fashion, I discovered there were sensible rules about how to use color and shape to emphasize and deemphasize your figure in all the right ways. I was a web designer with some graphic design classes in my past, so many of the ideas resonated with concepts I'd learned in college. I wanted to use this knowledge to show off my new body, like polishing a brand-new car for all the neighbors to see.

What I hadn't consciously realized about fashion was that what you wear affects how you feel. As a child I understood this instinctively when I raided our box of dress-up clothes. In the box were karate outfits my mother had bought in Japan on the long way home around the world after her stint in the Peace Corps. Instantly they would transform me from a wimpy grade-schooler into a stealthy ninja. An old peach nightgown became an elegant dress I'd wear to a cocktail party. My favorite item was the sparkly silver cape with metallic threads fraying around the edges. It was made of material popular only among beauty pageant contestants, but it turned me into a princess. I doubt any real princess would be caught wearing something so tacky, but it didn't matter. The clothes made me feel like a princess even if I looked like a pretender to the throne.

Fat-girl clothes never made me feel pretty. I would wear clothes that were too big for me, thinking they'd hide the fat when in reality they only made me look larger than I was. I couldn't find clothes that made me feel half as good as that cheap cape had. It might sound trivial to be complaining about not being allowed to shop at regular clothing stores, but being shut out from buying clothes at trendy shops was like being told, "You don't deserve to feel pretty. You can't be sexy. You don't get to be human."

This had a cyclical effect on my size because when I felt bad about myself, I would eat, which would make me fatter, which would make me feel bad about myself again. It was the fat-girl cycle of life. I once read an opinion article claiming it was bad that new plus-size retailers were offering better clothing than had been previously available, arguing that if fat people could find nice clothes, they wouldn't try to get thin. I found this logic flawed. Frequently people who want to lose weight will bash themselves, but it's only when you think you are worth the effort of self-improvement that you have a chance of succeeding. Wearing pretty clothes helped me feel better about myself. It made me feel as if I were a person worthy of losing weight. When I felt ugly in my baggy 4X pants, I wanted to devour ice cream sandwiches. If anything, fat people deserved good-looking clothes more than anyone else because we needed them more. Did skinny people want us to be fat *and* poorly dressed? Or should we just go around naked?

Now that I was shopping at new stores, I had to figure out the terrain. I had usually just headed for the fat clothes and kept my head down. A couple of months earlier, a department store had been having a 40-percent-off sale (also known as the "we've been bought by our competitor and need to dump this merchandise quick" sale). It was a typical department store and as with any typical department store, I didn't shop there. My salary was not fat enough to justify spending $80 on a sweater. I *had* spent most of my life fat enough not to fit into most of the clothes it sold. But it was 40 percent off already marked-down items! I decided to go to show off the fact that I could now walk around the mall from the far end of the parking lot without requiring CPR.

I had a lot of goals in life, but the one that seemed to come up the most frequently was "Don't look stupid!" I was reminded of this when I ventured into the store. Whenever entering unknown retail territory, I first surreptitiously assessed the layout of the store without giving away the fact that I had no clue where I was going. Even if I were wandering through the petites' section, I tried to walk confidently as if to say, "Why, yes, I am a big, tall, fat girl, but I am walking through the petite section *on purpose*. So there!" I sometimes prepared an excuse in case anyone stopped me to help, usually that I was shopping for my tiny, imaginary sister, the same one I baked cakes for.

I also didn't want to appear low class by shopping in a section that I clearly didn't belong in. When I had vacationed in New York (my college graduation present), somewhere along the walk between my hotel and Central Park I stumbled into a Bloomingdale's to pee. After using the restroom, I sat down on a black, padded couch in the misses' section to rest. I gazed up at the slender white mannequins with empty faces wearing tank tops that would barely fit around my thighs. I felt so out of place that I feared security might actually kick me out, if they were strong enough to haul my huge body out the door. I clearly didn't belong there among the thin and glamorous women of New York. I was a pauper stopping by to use the king's gold-plated bathroom. It wouldn't have mattered if I were richer than God. I felt out of my class.

When I was wandering around department stores, I'd usually end up in the right section by chance. I used to get very confused because I didn't understand the differences between women's, misses', juniors', and petite sizes. If something was a size Large I didn't know how large that was until I was alone in a dressing room. This led to paranoia as I was browsing the racks. I didn't want to be seen clearly browsing the wrong section, causing people to wonder, *What is* she *doing shopping in that section?* I don't know why I thought anyone was interested in what part of the store I was shopping in. I didn't care what racks other people were browsing.

I was amazed at the sheer quantity of clothing that department stores stocked. It was enough to clothe all of Luxembourg. I was used to being restricted to the little corner marked off for plus-sizes. There were so many clothes to sort through, so many stores to explore. I had to start putting thought into what I would buy instead of just buying whatever looked best at Lane Bryant. For the first time in my adult life, clothes were making me happy. I bought a pink pajama top decorated with hearts and cutesy skulls and crossbones that made me smile every time I wore it while brushing my teeth. Good clothing injected tiny moments of joy into my life at the most unexpected times.

But I was also disappointed to discover that not every piece of clothing I touched would magically fit me. The misses' section had looked like the land of milk and honey when I hadn't been drinking skim milk. I thought if I got small enough to shop over there, I'd never have trouble finding clothes again. Too bad this wasn't true. While my hunting grounds were greatly expanded, some items rode up over my belly button or hung off my shoulders. I discovered that clothes that were labeled the same size could be differently sized and cut, especially if they were from different clothing lines.

I wonder if when the industrial revolution enabled the proliferation of ready-to-wear clothing, the inventors of standardized sizing had any inkling of the psychological horrors they were unleashing upon women. Mass-produced clothing may save time spent over a sewing machine, but the true price is found on that number inside the garment, not on the price tag. Clothing is cut for an imaginary hypothetical woman, yet every woman has an unordinary feature. We are left trying to squeeze our atypical butts or boobs into a standardized package.

Like your age, size may be nothing more than a number. But like any symbol, numbers have as much power as we give them. A size 10 seems so much worse than a size 8 because it requires two digits instead of one. It's the same mind manipulation that makes the $19.99 shoes seem such a better bargain than a $20 pair. My mother worked as a seamstress in a bridal store, where she witnessed radical emotional changes induced by numbers. Tears of defeat or exclamations of joy, all because of a digit or two. She has suggested there would be a good niche market for an entrepreneur who replaced the sizing tags in dresses with smaller numbers.

The most frustrating thing about women's sizing is that it doesn't mean anything. When you buy a pair of size 28-jeans, shouldn't they measure 28 of something? They're not 28 inches or 28 centimeters, not a measure of circumference or length, not the number of tears you'll shed when learning your size. It's just a 28. And one clothing line's 28 may not even be the same size as another's.

The National Bureau of Standards conducted a sizing survey of women between 1949 and 1952, taking fifty-seven different body measurements of thousands of American women.[2] In 1958 the standards were published after being accepted by the industry, but eventually the average woman's shape changed as obesity proliferated. Some manufacturers started labeling their larger sizes with smaller numbers, a technique called vanity sizing. A common factoid of hope passed around by fat girls is that Marilyn Monroe was a size 14. Sadly, this was a size 14 from my mother's day, not mine, which means I would never have bumped into Norma Jean at Lane Bryant.

These standardized sizes are used today only for clothes patterns available at sewing stores. When I watched far too much *Project Runway* and decided I too could sew, I was in for a surprise that had nothing to do with how much suede costs. I pulled out a pattern for a wrap top from the neatly organized metal drawer at my local sewing supply shop to discover I was a 20. I'd lost almost 200 pounds by that point and I was a 20? By that time I was down to medium or a 12 in most stores. Maybe this was why more women didn't sew.

I suppose that there must have been a time between the moment I was cut out of my mother's womb and when I neared the four-hundred mark that I fit into these smaller sizes. I just couldn't remember when. I was so proud of wearing size Large shirts that I posted a picture of myself standing next to my new car on my blog, which had some regular readers now. When I was obese, I probably would have just posted a picture of the car sans owner. While everyone loved the shiny new addition to my debt, a reader named Susan summed up the consensus well with her comment, "If you had on pants that were the right size, we would have all been even more impressed."

Evidently my jeans were as baggy as MC Hammer's balloon pants. I was a tube top away from getting arrested by the fashion police. I rehabilitated myself, ditching the size-26 jeans for the next size down, snapped another photo, and posted it, certain that I would win the approval of my readers. Instead I got this comment from M, "Those pants? Do not fit you either. And your shirt is too big."

Now my entire outfit was under criticism. I slept on it, wondering if I were in denial about my size. If I went shopping in Chicago, would I be one of those poor saps pulled aside by the *Oprah* makeover crew to do a show on what not to wear? As I moved my laundry basket the next morning, I saw the box of skinny clothes in the closet sitting beneath it. Trying on old jeans and blouses had been one of the best ways for me to determine how fat I was during different times of my life. I pulled open the cardboard lid and looked inside at the old shirts and pants that I'd outgrown but could never bring myself to throw out, always holding out hope I might be thin one day. I sorted through old clothes and memories. That was the brown shirt I wore around campus my freshman year of college. Those were the black, checked shorts I lived in at summer camp in 1997. Why did I ever think cargo pants were appropriate for temp work?

I pulled out the old corduroys that had been my dream pants. When I'd lost weight after high school one of my goals was to be able to wear these pants. I'd bought them when I was sixteen. They'd only just barely fit then and they had never fit again.

I tried them on and they fit. Really fit. I could stand and sit down in them without inhaling half the oxygen in the room. They were a size

22. I *was* in denial about the pants. My blog readers might have been confrontational, but they were right. I couldn't fit into the corduroys when I weighed 220 in college, but I could when I weighed 229 now. I must have developed muscle after all. I had completely missed the stage in my life when I was a size 24. It was like waking up from a coma and losing one year of my life.

I kept losing weight until I saw the brown bottom of the box of skinny clothes. It hadn't seen the light of day for more than a decade.

CHAPTER 10

Two Weddings and a Funeral

Fat girls of the world, please forgive me. I fulfilled a fat-girl stereotype at my aunt's wedding reception. I stole a piece of cake.

That's a lie. I stole two pieces of cake.

I did not get caught. That would have set back the fat girl acceptance movement by several years. I was sneaky and avoided capture, so I set us back only by a few weeks, or at most a month or two.

I was somewhat exhausted from attending my second wedding in two weeks and making conversation at a table with a couple of aunts, an uncle, and two first cousins once removed. My aunt had gotten two bites into her apple spice cake before she got up to snatch a slice of the armadillo cake from a passing waiter. It wasn't made from armadillo, just shaped like one as a tribute to the film *Steel Magnolias*. A couple of cuts with the cake knife revealed red velvet filling inside the pastry mammal, which made it look like a bleeding sacrifice to the marriage gods. Then the DJ started spinning *YMCA* by the Village People and everyone at the table headed to the dance floor, leaving their food unguarded around a woman who'd lost more than a hundred pounds.

It was a huge tactical error.

I was halfway through my own slice of apple spice cake when I had already decided I wanted another. I wished scientists could figure out how to stimulate the proper neurons in my brain to re-create this taste experience. Then I could enjoy it without actually consuming calories. It would be like birth control for food, all the pleasure and none of the possible negative side effects. Sadly the slices were pretty small, only two-thirds the size of a slice of bread, so the pleasure of eating them didn't last long. As I stared at my aunt's unguarded piece of cake, I was stuck in a moral quandary. *She must not want that fine culinary creation,* I thought. *She got a different piece instead. It would be a shame to waste a piece of cake. It would make baby Jesus cry.* For purely religious reasons, I leapt up, snatched the plate, devoured the cake, and shoved the empty plate onto my uncle's place setting. Fat girl's first rule of stealing food: Always get rid of the evidence. Second rule: If necessary, frame someone else.

Baby Jesus must have been really happy that I didn't make him cry because my younger brother, Jim, came over from the adjoining table with another slice of apple spice cake. Jesus was multiplying the cake like loaves of bread and fish. Jim had grabbed the icy wedge from my diabetic cousin who couldn't eat cake. I felt so horrible for her that I scarfed down the entire slice and licked all the crumbs so there was nothing left to tempt her.

As the DJ kept spinning hokey tunes people liked dancing to only at weddings, the servers swooped in and completely cleared our table before anyone sprained his or her back doing the bunny hop. They took all the plates, even the ones full of food. All evidence of my stolen cake was removed from the scene of the crime, and I hadn't even needed to bribe anyone. My grand theft pastry was completed flawlessly. I didn't even feel bad about eating it. I didn't want to be a woman who never took pleasure in food without feeling guilty. I didn't feel bad about stealing it either, but that was because I had questionable ethics. Cake that good was hard to regret. I could get hit by a bus any day. It was best to enjoy life and good food while I could. My weight loss was a cross-country trip, not a race across town. I had to stop and check out the world's largest ball of twine and the giant dinosaur statue on the way. Who wanted to stay cooped up in the car the whole time?

Besides, I had been brave enough to attend both weddings in sleeveless dresses that brazenly displayed my batwings of underarm flab. I deserved a reward, especially for not swinging my arms too wide and accidentally smacking a kid in the eye by doing the Macarena. I'd decided to buy two formal dresses for the weddings, because even though I was wearing a size-14 dress, I felt great about myself. The last time I'd been to a wedding, I had been a bridesmaid in a size-26 gown. I was paired with a groomsman whose posture was so good I was tempted to refer him to a proctologist who could check for a flagpole up his ass. I felt like a blob rolling down the aisle next to him.

I'd started dress hunting when my mother brought home the spring catalog from the bridal store where she worked. That was when I realized a frightening truth—most formal dresses were sleeveless. There were literally only two dresses with sleeves featured in thirty-six pages of designs. At first I thought this was because the store was targeting skinny girls. The designers obviously didn't realize that fat girls hated their flabby upper arms. As I continued my search for plus-size dresses online, I discovered this was not just skinny-girl couture. Sleeves were out. Some dresses came with a wrap to drape around the wearer's arms, but I knew I would fidget with it all night long or accidentally dip the end in the toilet. I pitied anyone who had a scar on her shoulder or a mutant mole on her arm that she didn't want to display.

I visited a local plus-size thrift store in hopes of finding something beautiful and cheap. I discovered a silver dress with sparkly straps and took it into the makeshift dressing room that doubled as a bathroom. I pulled it on over my purple panties and mismatched bra, twisting my arm like I was trying to get myself to say "uncle" as I zipped it up the back. I turned to look in the mirror.

Sleeves were overrated. This was the dress. No one cared as much about my underarm flab as I did anyway.

It was only a couple of weeks later that I had to shop for a funeral.

My father's sister in New Jersey had terminal cancer. My life was just beginning again, but hers was near the end. I walked into my favorite clothing store and started circling the racks like a vulture, searching for something black. It felt wrong to be shopping for the funeral of a woman who wasn't even dead yet. The beeping of the register at the moment the cashier rung up my black polyester pants felt like the final death knell, as if the act of buying the clothes might kill her from a thousand miles away. I had the pants, so I had better have a funeral to wear them to.

By the next Wednesday I was driving out to New Jersey from Indiana with my younger brother. I had planned on packing boxes that day in preparation for the move out of my mother's house and into my new apartment, but I had no grounds to complain about rescheduling my U-Haul reservations. My mother was still alive, after all, even if I felt half dead from all the cake stealing and small talking I'd done earlier in the month.

I would also get to see my father for the first time since the day we'd stood in the Johnson County courthouse and witnessed the official dissolution of my parents' marriage. Two weddings and a funeral all in one month. If I crashed two more weddings would Hugh Grant show up to seduce me?

I hadn't made any long-distance trips since I'd starting eating right. I stocked a cooler full of celery sticks, apples, and oranges as a defense against fast food. If we careened off a cliff and became trapped in the twisted metal of our wrecked car, we'd have survival food for a week. I ate a salad at each rest break (though eating a burger and fries would have been much more convenient) because salads were preferable to grilling chicken breasts on the engine block.

After twelve hours on the road, we stumbled past two rabbits and a cat into my aunt and uncle's back kitchen door in Wilmington, Delaware. After depositing our bags in the guest rooms, I wandered back to the kitchen, where a wall of casseroles and baked goods lined the counter like the Great Wall of Carbohydrates.

"Are you hungry? Do you want something to drink?" my aunt Beth asked.

"Oh, we just ate a couple of hours ago. I'm not that hungry," I replied, hovering at the counter. I really wasn't hungry. I hoped she didn't think I was secretly starving but lying about it. When I had been fat I didn't want people to think all I did was eat, but now that I was managing my weight I didn't want people to think all I did was not eat.

"Are you sure?" Beth asked as she leaned over to open the oven and pull out . . . a fruit salad. "The church ladies have been ringing the doorbell all day. We've got brownies, pies, turkey . . ."

"Is that a baked fruit salad or something?" I replied. The water in Wilmington was polluted by all the chemical plants nearby, but did they have to cook every food they washed?

Beth laughed. "Oh, no! When I'm not using the oven to cook I sometimes use it for storage. Do you want some?" She set the salad on the kitchen table.

"No, that's okay." Beth seemed worried that they'd never be able to eat all this food before it went bad. I doubted it would all fit in their fridge. It did seem strange that the price of admission to a house of mourning was baked goods. Didn't people usually *lose* their appetites when they were in bereavement? Did visitors leave brownies lying around in the hopes that the scent of chocolate would tempt mourners to eat?

The next day my aunt and uncle, two cousins, my brother, and I drove to the viewing in their van. When I entered the long lobby that stretched the length of the building, I saw a bearded man in a black suit at the end of the hallway who resembled my father—if he had lost ninety pounds. I waved halfheartedly at the man, unsure if he were my dad, not wanting to commit too hard to the gesture in case I'd made a mistake. I could always claim I'd been swatting a mosquito.

The man bounded forward down the hall and his face came into focus. It *was* my father. "Hello!" he said warmly, smiling, glad to see me after so many years. I was surprised by how different he looked. I bet this was how old friends felt when they saw me again. I wondered what he thought of my own transformation.

"Hi," I said awkwardly. We stared at each other. The eye contact made me uncomfortable. We hadn't talked much since he'd left three years ago, and I didn't know where to start. Someone said something eventually and we ventured into the viewing room. Between the first and second viewing the family decided to go to an Italian restaurant. I stood in the faux fresco lobby next to my dad waiting for the servers to push enough tables together to seat us all.

"So, you've been dieting, eh?" he asked me.

"Yeah, sort of," I replied. "Eating more fruits, veggies, and lean meats. Stuff like that."

"Do you count calories?" he asked. "I try to keep it under 1,600 calories a day," he said pulling out a small notebook to show me his food diary.

"Not really," I said. "I keep track of what I've eaten in my head and sort of guesstimate." It was far too uncomfortable to talk about why he'd left, but we could talk about calories. That was . . . nice?

"I found your blog, by the way," he said.

I paused in fear. "Oh, which one?" I asked. I irregularly posted to a personal journal, but I'd been writing in the fat blog three or four times a week lately.

"PastaQueen.com, the weight-loss blog."

Only the solemnity of the occasion kept me from slapping my hands to my cheeks and imitating the Edvard Munch painting, *The Scream*. There should be a word for the feeling of fear and horror when you realize a family member has discovered your blog. Emblogessment, perhaps? I suddenly tried to remember the content of every one of my two hundred entries in the span of two seconds. *Had I said anything about him?*

"Oh," I eeped.

"It's a great site. I'm really proud of you."

"Thanks," I said. *Had he told anyone else about this?*

Our party name was called. Our table was ready. I was rescued from the 212th awkward conversation that month. Only eighty-six or so more to go. I was starting to build up a tolerance.

After the viewing I said bye to my dad. The rest of us returned to my aunt and uncle's house and congregated around the kitchen table, where cheesecake, cracker boxes, and liquor bottles were piled high like a barrier against the bad feelings. They wouldn't have to cook for weeks. The day before I had barely snacked on any of the chocolates or cookies, though I did eat a slice of cheese because I didn't want to be viewed as "the girl on a diet" who wouldn't eat. That was like being the prudish girl who wouldn't drink and go dancing. But now I was hungry and tired and had cheesecake clinging to the roof of my mouth. We talked for hours.

Beth leaned back in the wooden kitchen chair and wondered out loud, "Why do we always end up entertaining guests in the kitchen?

We've got a huge living room we never use." I spread some cheese on a cracker, but I didn't say anything. The kitchen is the heart of the home. Where else would we spend an evening of mourning?

On the way back to Indiana I ate more salads. I was starting to get sick of radicchio and restaurants that were out of fat-free salad dressing packets, but I didn't want to stray too far from my plan. If I ate one Big Mac, I might regain all 150 pounds right there in the front seat. That could really affect our gas mileage. A piece of cake stolen here and there was fine, but I didn't want to relearn my bad eating habits. It had been stressful not knowing when or where I would be eating or if there would be any carrots on the buffet table next to the potato salad and fried chicken wings. I was completely out of my routine.

My only good exercise had been walking twenty blocks around Washington DC with an old high school friend. I matched her fast walking pace so well that I kept stepping on her flip flops. I wondered if my concern about food and exercise could be considered an obsession. I didn't want to break my number one rule: Don't get crazy. But if I didn't catch small slips when they happened I was bound to get fat again. I liked my new ass far too much to let that happen.

We arrived back home Saturday night, and I spent Sunday recuperating. I weighed in and was happy to see I was up only half a pound. I tried packing up the last of my stuff for my rescheduled move on Monday, but ended up napping on the couch instead. I was still digesting all the apple spice cake from the wedding, cheesecake from the wake, and too many buttery Bob Evans biscuits from our final dinner stop.

The next morning, I got my mother, Jim, and his muscular friend Wes to load the rental truck as I drove ahead to my new apartment complex to sign the lease. The rental manager showed me my unit for approval. Looking at the closed doors of my new neighbors in the courtyard, I was happy that no one here would know that I had been morbidly obese. The last time I'd made an identity change like this was when we'd moved to Maryland in the first grade and I'd stopped going by the nickname Jenny. Only the postman might profile me as a fat girl when he stuffed my Lane Bryant catalogs into the mailbox.

I'd requested a unit on the second floor so I could incorporate more incidental exercise into my life when I trampled up and down the stairs carrying groceries or hauled a basket of dirty clothes to the laundry room. The complex was also close to a nature trail that stretched through the city on a former railway line. I wanted to get off my treadmill and run outside. The complex had a small exercise room with an elliptical trainer that I wanted to try too. I was now making decisions about where I would live based on the exercise options the location provided. I wasn't just brainwashed into a life of fitness, I was brainwashed, rinsed, and dried.

The van containing all my earthly possessions arrived in the parking lot. We bounded up and down the stairs carrying boxes of books and CDs. The last year and a half of running and eating well had all been leading up to this. Some people train for marathons, but if you know anyone who is moving, it would be more practical to train for that. You could fill up cardboard boxes with free weights and walk up and down several flights of stairs. Rearrange all the furniture in your living room. Then move it back. The day after my move I had so many bruises on my forearms from carrying boxes that I looked like I was in a violent relationship.

Someone should start a service in which instead of wasting money on gym memberships, you volunteer to help people move. You'd get a cardio workout, and you'd actually be accomplishing something instead of just wearing down the soles of your running shoes. It would be a blend of community service and exercise. You could start by doing first-floor moves and then work your way up to sixth-floor apartments with no elevators.

I typically prided myself on being a big strong woman who could carry her own groceries and squash her own bugs, but I did have limits. I let the men shift the heavy piece of machinery known as my treadmill up the stairs. I bought them a case of beer in payment.

By the end of the day, I'd thanked my family and sent them away. I shoved a bowl of cat food under the bed where my kitty was cowering from posttraumatic stress and realized I'd barely eaten all day myself. When I kept my mind busy, I didn't notice when I was hungry. I'd had a sandwich for breakfast, a chocolate-chip cookie dough milk shake for lunch, and a salad for dinner. I didn't have much of an appetite. I'd forced myself to chew the last piece of tomato in yet another salad only because I didn't want to become someone who tried to subsist on eight hundred calories a day and collapsed because all her muscle had been metabolized. How would I carry my lamps up the stairs then?

My new refrigerator was as cold and barren as the Siberian tundra. It contained only three cups of yogurt, two cheese sticks, half a two-liter of Diet Dr. Pepper, and an unused packet of Italian dressing. By the end of the night I was wishing I'd packed that bottle of rum my mom had offered from the cupboard. I'd turned it down because alcohol contains so many empty calories, but it sounded pretty good right about now. My cooking skills were momentarily useless because I didn't own a microwave and wouldn't let myself buy one until I unearthed my 20-percent-off coupon, which was buried in one of the boxes that created a geodesic garden in my living room. Cardboard was high in fiber, right? I could eat and unpack at the same time.

I ventured to the closest grocery store to stock my fridge and was frustrated that I'd have to learn a new store layout. I'd finally figured out where every item I liked was located at my old store, and now I was playing dodge-the-salami. It didn't even carry my favorite brand of fudgsicles. I had to stock my entire kitchen, so I bought more food than I'd ever bought in my life, filling my cart to capacity.

When I finally dug the scale out from one of my boxes, I was not surprised to learn I'd lost five pounds, probably because of dehydration and the near toxic levels of stress I'd been under the past week. I weighed my cat a couple of weeks later and discovered he'd lost a pound too, mainly because of the hide-under-the-bed diet. That might work for me too, but it would freak out my friends and relatives.

A big part of my life had been dedicated to weight loss lately. I considered it to be my hobby, but no matter how much I wanted to focus on dropping more weight, life insisted on carrying on around me. People would always be getting married, dying, and moving—though I hoped they'd stop doing it all in the same month. I had sometimes thought it would be nice to lock myself away on a fat farm where all my food and exercise could be controlled, but I preferred living in the real world, even if that involved tempting platters of chocolate-chip cheesecake served with a very good excuse to eat it. I'd indulged in some sweets, but I hadn't gorged myself under the pressure, and I'd eaten as best I could under the circumstances. I soon returned to my exercise routine with barely a hiccup. I'd survived a stressful month without seeking comfort in food.

I returned to work on Tuesday and sat at my desk with my eyes unfocused, as if I were gazing through the screen trying to see a magic 3-D photo print. I'd just had six days off from work.

I needed a vacation.

CHAPTER 11

Trail Mix

"**E**xcuse me, are you walking your cat?"

The man I'd asked this question of looked up from the foliage on the side of the paved trail. A tan tabby cat was walking four yards ahead of him, sniffing flowers and stomping on bugs. His owner meandered slowly behind, no leash in hand.

"Yes, I am," he replied, hands in his pockets, completely unfazed by my question.

"That's *awesome*," I told him as I let the chain-link gate close. I walked back to my apartment complex.

I was madly in love with the long path and its red line running down the middle. It was part of the new life in my new apartment, a life in which people walked cats instead of dogs. I might have to start eating out of the dumpster to afford the rent, but banana peels were high in fiber. The day after my move, I glimpsed runners, bikers, and in-line skaters whizzing along as I drove home from work. I imagined they were calling out to me, "Come with us! Frolic among the trees and flowers like pixies while elevating your heart rate for long intervals at a time!" I drove on instead, telling myself I really needed to buy a microwave before the store closed at nine. This was true, but I was also putting off my inaugural run because I'd never exercised in front of other people. I'd used the treadmill in the privacy of my own home because I didn't want to be the gross obese girl at the gym. As a fat person I probably had more of a right to the gym than anyone else. I obviously needed it more. Unfortunately, that argument never got me to the Stairmaster.

I convinced myself to tie up my running shoes after I repeated an old saying: You wouldn't care about what other people think of you if you knew how infrequently they do. In other words, "Everyone else is a self-centered bastard too." It was easy for me to assume anyone in visual range of my arms was thinking, "If she flaps her elbows hard enough she could fly away." It was more likely that they pedaled by thinking, "My panties are really bunching up in these shorts." Even if they did spare a moment to think disparaging thoughts about me, it was just a passing blip between gear changes.

I waited for a week before I put on my sweatpants, sports bra, and T-shirt to go for a walk. I checked that my apartment key was in my pocket and pulled the door closed behind me. I turned and ran smack into a pack of thin girls leaving the apartment two doors down. Given the choice between running into a pack of thin girls and a pack of wolves, I hesitated a bit longer than any rational human being should. How big were the wolves? Had they eaten recently? How about the thin girls?

I had been feeling so good about myself lately that I imagined a groovy theme song playing in the background as I strode confidently down the street. But if I encountered a pack of thinner, prettier girls, my theme song came to a screeching halt. *Don't be intimidated,* I told myself. *They are not better than you just because they have 15 percent body fat and skin as smooth as goat's milk. Yak's milk is what it's all about this year.*

I waved hello to them as I rushed down the stairs, chiding myself for being ridiculous. The pack consisted of friends of the neighbor who had been the nicest to me. She'd said hello every time I'd seen her and offered to help me carry empty boxes to the dumpster. The only person she was competing with in the Nice Neighbor Pageant was Bill from downstairs. I didn't see him often, which was probably for the best since he would have been killed if he'd walked out his door when my two-liter of Sprite Zero rolled off the balcony. Everyone else in the complex had been aloof. If I was still morbidly obese, I would have attributed it to fat discrimination. Now I just knew they were rude.

I had no reason to fear this girl or her friends. So what if they liked to lie around the pool and display their gorgeous bodies for the whole complex? I wondered if female rivalry were hard-coded into our genes as a way for us to get the best mates. It was the early Darwin alert system, "Warning! Rival, rival! Endangering chances of procreation!" I hoped it was genetics because I hated to think I was a shallow, jealous person. Blaming the inescapable forces of nature was better than acknowledging possible character flaws.

I had lots of reasons to lose weight. One of them was to become more attractive to men, but I also wanted to stop feeling inferior around other women. Men weren't as picky as they pretended to be. My mom's bridal store sold dresses all the way up to size 26, so fat girls were definitely getting married and getting laid, even if they were harder to carry over the threshold. Being thin was often a competition between women in which the losers were awarded the parting gifts of envy and an inferiority complex. I had a couple of thin, hot female friends who were on the receiving end of this type of jealousy and I knew they didn't deserve it. Just because you could post a picture of yourself on your blog and get thirty "OMG, u r so hot!" comments in an hour didn't mean you weren't also intelligent and thoughtful. You could have big boobs and a big brain. Fat or thin, pretty or homely, was there ever a winning team?

After escaping the thin girls, I made it to the gate leading to the trail. I took three steps across the gravel and landed on the path. It was the middle of summer, so the trail was as crowded as an electronics store on Black Friday. I chose a direction and started walking.

"On your left!" someone called out behind me. I turned around and nearly underwent a rhinoplasty when a man in Lycra bike shorts and a sports jersey whizzed past me hunched over a bicycle. "On your left" must be secret trail talk for "Move your ass to the right, slowpoke!" I was glad I had stuck emergency contact information in my pocket along with my key. It was rush hour out here. I wouldn't have been surprised if I had found a body on the side of the trail with a skid mark up its back. A girl in jean shorts and a tank top skated past me, keys held out like a weapon in one hand while she gabbed on the cell phone in her other. I hoped she wouldn't collide with the father pushing a stroller and puncture her lung on her keys. At least they'd be able to call 911 right away.

During the next few days I saw an amazing array of contraptions traveling on the trail. It felt like an exhibition at the World's Fair. A woman rode a bike with a small tent-like trailer attached to the back and a toddler inside. A middle-aged man wearing a sweatband was making good time on a huge tricycle that he reclined in like a lounge chair. I had not yet seen anyone on a unicycle, but there had been Segways and a man on a penny-farthing bicycle, a contraption with a front wheel as large as a tractor's and a back wheel the size of a skateboard's.

It was as if I'd entered the lobby of a casting agency without traveling to L.A. A young woman Rollerbladed by holding a fluffy white poodle in her arms. An elderly couple enjoying the fresh air were the only people walking more slowly than me. A woman ran past me with a severe wobble in her walk. I didn't know if she were practicing a cutting-edge exercise technique or if she were disabled. I later learned she was a competitive walker. Some teenage girls passed me in the other direction in dresses and heels, probably headed to the village district's shops and restaurants. A muscular man jogged by in the other direction. My eyes lingered. I did love studying all the natural specimens out here among nature.

I picked up my pace and became breathless. I was worried my downstairs neighbor would complain if I used my treadmill too much, so I wanted to run outside more often. Running outside was harder than running on the treadmill. I had no idea how fast I was going or how far I had run. The stone markers appeared only every half mile. Had I become less fit during my travels and moving adventures? When I checked the time on my watch, I realized I was running much faster than I had been inside. Of course I was winded. This might have been why I had never run an entire mile nonstop as a kid; I wasn't pacing myself correctly. The jogger in front of me slowed down to a walk. I trundled past him as fast as my chubby legs would take me. Twenty seconds later he passed me on the left. That was a rather short break. Maybe he didn't like being lapped by the fat girl.

I took a "look, but don't speak" approach to the trail. I made brief eye contact with others to be polite and to ward off possible assailants, but I never talked to anyone. On my fourth day, one of the other runners stopped acting like a cardboard cutout and actually spoke to me. I was stopped at the crosswalk on my way home, wondering how many hours of my life had been wasted waiting at red lights, when a thirtysomething man with sweaty hair crossed against the light. "It's kind of a hot day for it, but you're doing well!" he commented. I looked behind me expecting to see someone more athletic standing behind me. There was no one there. I half-nodded at the man as he jogged off. Conversations on the trail seemed to be hit-and-runs. People shouted something out quickly and then ran in the other direction, like a game of tag with words.

The light changed and I started to think about what he'd said. Someone was commending me for the effort I put forth exercising and seemed inspired by it. Why was that so inspiring? I hadn't heard him complimenting everyone he ran past, only me. Just because I was fat didn't mean I needed to be coddled. It wasn't even that hot, maybe seventy-five degrees on the mostly shaded path. If we lived in Texas this would be a chilly summer afternoon. I shook my head as I breathed the humid air deeply. I was overanalyzing. I should just take it as a compliment and be grateful he didn't say, "Move over, fatty!"

After a fifty-year-old man ran by me wearing nothing but a pair of tiny gym shorts from the eighties and a sweaty chest full of hair, I decided it was okay to wear a tank top.

I had a dark blue tank top embroidered with Eeyore, the donkey from *Winnie the Pooh.* "Thanks for noticing me" was a good motto for the invisible girl. It was a size medium. I'd bought it when I was at my lowest weight at the beginning of college and even then it had been too tight to wear without outlining my nipples. Now it fit snugly but comfortably. More important, it made me feel cuter than kittens in a bathroom sink.

I felt a surge of energy and decided to sprint down the trail. I stopped at the crosswalk and noticed a guy on a bike in his late thirties with a scraggly beard, no shirt, and a bit of a belly. We made eye contact.

"That looks like a lot of fun," he said jokingly, referring to the heat and humidity.

"Oh, yeah," I faked laughter and pulled a sarcastic face.

"I wish I could do that. I just ride a bike," he replied.

I just nodded, my talent as the world's second-worst conversationalist behind a blind, mute boy in a coma revealed. The traffic stopped and I continued jogging. The biker guy passed me.

"Don't have too much fun!" he said as he rode past.

"Ha, I'll try not to!" I replied. Then he turned his head around and yelled, "And don't tell your boyfriend about me."

I imagine I paused in midstride, floating above the ground like Wile E. Coyote does before he realizes he's stepped off a cliff and plummets to the ground. Had a shirtless hippie just hit on me? I think he did. I nearly stopped in the middle of the crosswalk, but regained my senses and continued on. Otherwise the headline in tomorrow's papers would have read, "Girl is hit on and then hit by car."

Men didn't hit on me. This was something that happened to other women. Some fat girls could take control of a room like an expert politician, exuding charm and confidence and have men eating out of their chubby fingers. I was not one of them. I was the type who thought, "Do I need to make eye contact with these people or is my dress pattern similar enough to the wallpaper that I can blend into the wall?" New people scared me. I avoided them. Because I was a fat person, they avoided me in return.

A couple of years earlier I had been at a deli, buying a submarine sandwich drenched in far too much mayonnaise, when a man at the table near the counter tried to make conversation with me. I answered his remarks as briefly and politely as possible. It was only months later that I realized he had been hitting on me. It hadn't occurred to me at the time that a guy might be interested in someone as fat as I was. I'd never had a serious boyfriend and I'd never made an effort to find one. This probably meant I had intimacy issues or "trouble making friends," as my kindergarten teacher had put it, as though I were one bad childhood away from moving to a shack in Montana that I would leave only to mail letter bombs. I preferred to think it made me an independent woman who could survive on her own in the world and didn't mind going to the movies alone. Who wanted to share the popcorn anyway?

The guy who hit on me at the deli had been thin, which further confused me because I assumed I'd have to date a fat guy. I would have preferred to date a thin guy because I was a big fat hypocrite who did not find obese men attractive, but thin guys didn't usually go for fat girls, or if they did they were too ashamed to admit it. Some of my prettier, thinner friends would complain about the burden of their looks. They fended off unwanted advances by men at clubs and rolled their eyes at honking horns and hollering when they walked past busy streets. I sympathized with them and admitted that this must be a problem, but it was a problem in the same way that filing taxes must be a pain for a millionaire who has to keep track of dividends and real estate deals and yacht purchases. It seemed like a damned good problem to have.

It might soon be my problem as well. I had just weighed in at below one hundred kilograms, which would have been a huge milestone if I lived in a country that used the metric system. In America this just meant I weighed about 220 pounds. My rate of loss had slowed down from the exciting ten pounds a month of the first year to a more reasonable five pounds a month. I was looking forward to hitting 202 pounds. Then I would cross the line between being obese and being overweight, according to the body mass index gurus. I knew this was just an arbitrary line created when you plugged my height and weight into an equation, but I wanted to be officially overweight instead of obese anyway. No doubt I would fluctuate up and down depending on how much I had to drink that day and when my last trip to the bathroom was. It would be like jumping back and forth over a state line.

But obese or overweight, it was now official. I was a sex object.

I heard the grocery store was a good place to pick up guys, but I decided it was a better place to pick up weird ingredients. The trail ran conveniently close to a grocery store, the post office, and the library. I was used to living in areas where I needed a car to complete errands, but now I could walk to places to accomplish the tasks of daily living without fear of being embedded in the grill of a passing Hummer. One evening I was bored with my standard recipes, so I browsed my healthy cookbooks for a new entrée. I picked out a tuna melt casserole that required something called milled flaxseed. I had no idea what flaxseed was and I didn't have a mill anyway, so I threw my backpack over my shoulder and walked a mile to the store. I was more thrilled than anyone shopping for flaxseed had a right to be. A year earlier I would never have been able to walk to the store without a dozen rest stops. I was achieving something other than just exercising my heart and lungs. I was on a quest for tuna casserole. When I pulled it out of the oven that evening, it tasted extra good, for reasons that had nothing to do with the seasonings.

That fall, when I needed to pick up some books on hold at the library, I calculated how far the walk was and figured I was fit enough to make the 5.25-mile round-trip. On the way back I recalled a blogger mentioning that she read books while walking home. I didn't know that was possible, just as I had been amazed by my friend who could knit while watching a movie with subtitles. I decided to take a page out of the blogger's book and started reading on my way back. It was surprisingly easy. I kept the red line down the middle of the concrete in my peripheral vision and watched out for doggy doo-doo.

My knees had been achy lately, probably permanently damaged from my years of obesity. I had intended to give them a break by walking the entire path instead of running. It continued to get darker. The path was much less crowded than usual. While it was nice that my chances of being run over by a biker were reduced, it also left a significant lack of witnesses if anyone decided to increase this summer's crime rate. I decided to jog the last half mile. There was nothing like the threat of rape and murder to push my exercise routine further. Fear elevated my heart rate in more ways than one.

When I wasn't checking over my shoulder for muggers hiding in the bushes, the trail was a calming place. I'd go there to let my thoughts wander like the leashed dogs I ran past. The disappearing sun was cutting into my meditation time. I ran in the evenings, and the lengthening fall days were shrinking my window of daylight. I wanted to write the sun a letter telling it to stop distancing itself and spending so much time with Australia. I wanted to make the most of our time together while the weather was still above freezing.

In an act of desperation, I tried running in the mornings. I was usually awake around dawn anyway, when my cat performed the Hokey Pokey on my face. He would put his left foot in (my eye), put his left foot out (on my neck), put his left foot in (my ear), and shake his tail in my face. It was surprisingly cold in the morning. The earth cooled off overnight and in the morning was still preheating to whatever the high temperature would be for that day. This did not stop some trail denizens from dressing like they were in Miami Beach. I was shivering in my pullover jacket and these people were jogging in shorts and sleeveless shirts. I heard running heated you up, but would it hurt to put on a pair of pants?

By lunchtime I felt as if I'd forgotten to fill up my gas tank before a cross-country trip. I'd walked four miles and I hadn't eaten enough afterward to compensate. The raspberry vodka my brother brought over the night before as an apology for eating my last piece of salmon might have had something to do with it too. I was exhausted, just like in the old days when I ate poorly and got the afternoon munchies. I did some stretches in my office to get my blood going. After a week, I decided morning running was not for me. The early bird may get the worm but the early worm deserved the bird.

I went for a run in the afternoon that weekend, a time much preferable to the crack of dawn. I was passing a water fountain when a blonde woman in a T-shirt stopped me.

"I was looking for a running partner," she said. "Is that something you would be interested in?" she asked.

Wow. Two years ago I could hardly walk around the mall without getting winded and now I was being solicited for my exercise prowess.

"I'm a slow runner too," she continued.

Oh. I was being solicited for my exercise inability. Still, it was an improvement. I was rather proud of my twelve-minute mile. It beat my fifteen-minute mile from high school. I thought about taking her up on her offer, but I looked at the changing leaves and felt the cool breeze and decided to turn her down. The seasons were changing, and I wouldn't be out here much until next spring. I felt bad since she had showed such courage in asking a stranger to be her partner.

"Sorry," I said and continued down the path slowly, but faster than I'd ever gone before.

On one of my last jogs down the trail I saw a 400-pound man in a motorized scooter on the dirt path that led to the riverbank. He was just sitting there as the joggers and bikers and in-line skaters whizzed by. I could probably attribute the crunching sound I heard to the breaking of twigs I was trampling over, but it might have been the sound of my heart breaking. Here was a man literally watching the world pass him by.

He was so large that I didn't doubt that he needed that vehicle to get around. He wasn't some hoodlum taking a grocery store scooter for a joy ride. I doubted he would have been able to walk a half mile without getting winded. I knew because I used to be almost as large as him. Back then, walking from a concert on the lawn at White River State Park to the zoo parking lot only half a mile away was my version of the Iron Man.

I didn't get a good look at him because I was actively attempting not to stare like he was a rare white tiger on exhibit at the zoo, but I was as drenched in pity as if I'd fallen off the bridge into the water. He looked so isolated even though he was surrounded by people. I wondered why he had come to the trail. Did he just want to be outside on a nice day like most of the people there? Had his battery died? I doubt he wanted my pity, but when I saw him I could only see my old fat self. I knew there wasn't anything I could do for the man. So I just kept running by, grateful that these days I was part of the world and not the one watching it pass by.

CHAPTER 12

I Should Know Better By Now

After losing 150 pounds, I felt like a dieting genius. Some days I felt so disciplined that it could rain chocolate chips like hail and I wouldn't bother catching the candies in my mouth. Other days, I wouldn't have minded the hail damage if it meant I had an excuse to devour a downpour of chocolate.

In May, just a month before I moved out, I had thoroughly searched the refrigerator for some cheese sticks, looking under every square packet of ketchup we'd seized from fast food restaurants. I couldn't find a speck of grated Parmesan, never mind an entire stick of mozzarella for my lunch bag. My mother or brother had probably eaten the last piece and hadn't told me. By three o'clock in the afternoon I was starving and ready to chomp on the chipboard laminate of my desk, so I decided to walk to the vending machine on the far side of the building instead.

The dieting gods might have been on my side when the vending machine down the hall from our office broke at the beginning of the year. The Snickers bars did seem to snicker at me as I walked to the ladies' room. My mother was hiding her ice cream under the frozen green beans at home, but I couldn't expect my coworkers to place a black veil over the vending machine's glass. After it stole one too many quarters from the employees, the malfunctioning machine was hauled off and never replaced.

However, there was another vending machine two floors down on the other side of the building. I didn't think it sold cheese sticks, but at least I would burn ten or twenty calories walking there. Out of all the sugar-soaked, carbohydrate-crammed items available, the animal crackers seemed to be the best choice. I dropped my eighty cents into the slot, entered my selection into the keypad, and . . . my crackers were pulled into a hostage situation with a dull wire coil. Ever since I saw an episode of *The West Wing* that claimed more people are killed each year by vending machines than by wolves, I'd been hesitant to rock or shake a machine to get an item. So, I inserted another eighty cents to get my crackers. As a bonus I also got the item that was right behind them: the Chips Ahoy Chocolate Chip Cookies.

It wasn't just raining chocolate chips, it was raining chocolate-chip cookies.

I ripped open the plastic bag and scarfed the cookies before I could find time to wonder how long they'd been sitting behind the herd of crackers. I could have left the cookies in the bin as a random act of kindness (unless the next customer was dieting too, in which case it would be a random act of meanness). But my philanthropic side was caught in a headlock with the money-conscious part of my brain, the part that had gotten me out of debt after two years of scrimping and saving. I didn't even know what "scrimping" meant, but I had done it. I couldn't deal with the fact that I would have wasted eighty entire cents if I didn't eat the cookies. I had an amazing ability to rationalize things I knew I shouldn't be doing.

If I had been prepared enough to bring breakfast, or if I'd had time before work to buy something to eat, I would never have gone to the vending machine in the first place. It was a chain reaction that started in the morning when I skipped breakfast and ended with a three-car pileup in front of the vending machine. The only real crash was the very real sugar crash I experienced an hour later. I was relieved I hadn't eaten my desk because I really wanted to take a nap on it. I felt crappy when I ate crap, not just from the guilt but from the food's effect on my body. It was difficult to remember how good I felt until I wasn't feeling that good. I needed the contrasts to remember.

Around the same time, boxes of cookies started showing up in the pantry of our house. When my mother decided to move to a two-bedroom apartment several years after the divorce, she had to clean out the attic, the basement, the two-car garage, the shed, the workshop, and the patio, sort through all the junk my father had left behind, and sell all the major appliances. After purging our possessions, she needed to binge. I would never be so cruel that I'd ask someone to stop buying chocolate, but I did ask her to keep it out of my sight. I had accepted I was weak willed when it came to certain foods; I just had to work around it. If I opened the freezer to unexpectedly stare down a tub of mint chocolate ice cream, it was like being mugged on the way to work. I wasn't expecting a battle, but now I had to put up a fight, dig fingernails into flesh. Most people recommend that you don't fight off muggers, just give them your wallet. Typically I wouldn't put up much of a fight with the ice cream either.

One day she left a package of Oreos on the shelf right above our garbage can. I snacked on two cookies in the short amount of time it took to turn over the blue plastic package and realize I'd just consumed seventy calories. That was more than a serving of my light yogurt, inhaled in less than a minute. I experienced the food equivalent of buyer's remorse, though I resisted the urge to toss my cookies.

Policemen are trained not to draw their guns unless they are prepared to use them. I decided I wouldn't bring any food into the house unless I was prepared to eat it.

It was strange living on my own again. I was a loner, but I still got lonely or bored sometimes. And here I was. Alone. In the apartment. With all the food. The only barrier between my newly decorated living room and the kitchen was a counter with bar stools. It took only six steps to grab a bowl of sugar-free pudding and two containers of fat-free vanilla yogurt topped with generous helpings of Go Lean Crunch. It was slightly reassuring that I pigged out on diet pudding instead of a pint of ice cream, but I'd still overeaten. I don't think those six steps burned off even a sixth of the calories I consumed. The food didn't fill the emptiness inside, either. I needed to keep busy. I could dress up my garden gnomes on the windowsill in Barbie clothes and put on a drag show for my She-Ra action figures. I could just go be bored on the trail instead of in my kitchen. Or I could attempt to accept that it was okay to feel alone or sad sometimes and that I didn't need to bury my face in a bowl of pudding to suffocate the feelings. I liked the sound of the drag show better.

The kitchen was also home to a dangerous appliance—the breadmaker. Years earlier when my mother had bought the white, rectangular box that hogged valuable real estate on the kitchen counter, I had laughed. I didn't see the point of buying a machine to make something that you could buy for a couple of dollars at the grocery store. But when I started dieting, I started making a loaf of whole grain bread every weekend. My mother was now the one laughing. The scent of freshly baked bread was better than any air freshener. I would snack on warm slices before the loaf had even cooled down.

I ate a lot of slices. Actually, I'd eat a whole loaf in a weekend. Whole grains can be good for you, but eating a toaster-size block of bread every weekend is probably too much of a good thing. When I lived with my family, they'd eat about a third of the loaf, but when I moved out I was doing all the digesting. Each time I told myself I wouldn't eat the whole thing, and then I'd do it anyway.

After the closing, my mother's Realtor gave her some gifts: bread, that the house may never know hunger; salt, that life may always have flavor; and wine, that joy and prosperity may reign forever. I don't know what she did with the salt, but she kept the wine and gave me the Hawaiian sweet bread mix. I *did* own the bread machine after all. I poured the powder into the metal mixing pan and then clicked it into the belly of the appliance. I would bake the bread and give it back to my mother. Of course I would. I was doing her a favor.

After my third slice, I decided I needed to evict the remaining bread from the apartment. Wrapping the loaf in a thin plastic produce bag and tying it firmly shut with a knot, I grabbed my car keys and hustled downstairs to the parking lot as if the bag's contents would explode at any moment. With a click of a button on my key ring, the trunk popped open and I tossed the bread into the back, next to my milk crate of spare oil and fix-a-flat. I slammed the trunk shut, imprisoning my great temptation so I wouldn't find myself idly cutting off a slice while it sat on the counter.

Then I left my car at the dealership across town.

I'd have to walk ten miles to eat the bread, which was just as likely as flying to Hawaii for a loaf. I hadn't intended to move it across town, but when my car stalled out at a stop sign, I left it overnight to be inspected and forgot about the bread. I didn't want to view food as dangerous, but there was no denying that some foods overrode the center of my brain that told me to stop eating when I was full. Normally my eating habits were similar to the action of the conveyor belt in the checkout line of the grocery store. It automatically scrolled forward until a box of oatmeal or a can of olives broke the infrared beam to stop the motion. Normally I would stop eating when the beam was tripped and I was full. When I ate bread, the beam in my mind didn't get tripped, and I wanted to keep eating and eating even though I knew I should switch off the conveyor belt shoving food into my mouth. I just couldn't find the off switch.

When I mentioned my bread problem on my blog, a reader named Ros came up with a brilliant solution that was obvious in its simplicity. "I keep it in the freezer and pop it in the toaster when I want it." Why hadn't I thought of that? Now I could eat bread that didn't smell like antifreeze.

A t the end of a long day, I dropped my purse in the hallway and entered the kitchen to feed my cat. I wondered if he'd noticed that I'd lost weight. There sure was less of me to curl up on. His tail started twitching as I peeled back the metal lid of his wet food. He kept poking his nose into the can as I scooped out the ground-up bits of animals that I didn't want to know the names of. I scraped all around the edges and whacked the remaining sticky clumps into the bowl with a few thumps.

And then I licked the spoon.

It was only when the meaty mess was sticking to the top of my mouth that I realized what I had done. All those years of licking the beaters clean of cake mix and scooping up wads of chocolate-chip cookie dough on the sly must have created an automatic response in my brain. I'd run down a well-beaten path in my neural pathways that said: Serve food, lick spoon.

Since it was already in my mouth, I figured I might as well swallow. This is a philosophy that I apply only to food. Surprisingly, the cat food didn't taste that bad. But I wasn't going to be making any cat food pâté recipes either. At least I had bought the diet variety.

I wondered how many other food choices in my life were made when I was on autopilot. There had been times when I'd grabbed a peppermint candy out of a dish on a receptionist's counter simply because it was there. I would usually finish all the food on my plate whether I was still hungry or not. When I ate at an Italian restaurant with my family, I told myself that just because the server put food in front of me didn't mean I had to eat it. Then I'd hide a slab of garlic bread in my stomach for safekeeping. I considered sneaking excess food onto my companions' plates when they weren't looking or throwing it at other patrons who were yapping on their phones too loudly.

At least I had a reasonable explanation for snacking on Savory Salmon with Hairball Control. It would have been a stretch convincing anyone it was an accident when I pigged out on an entire batch of apple cinnamon muffins. They were made with Splenda, which has zero calories but not zero guilt. Sitting at work, staring at the glare on my monitor, I thought, "I'm going to make muffins when I get home and eat far too many of them." And then I did. At least I had follow-through.

After I ate my muffins, I lay in bed with the painful feeling of being too full. I wished I was just at my goal already. Then a binge like this wouldn't be as bad. The muffins would have the same amount of calories whether I weighed 220 pounds or 160, but if I were just under my goal weight it would be like dipping into my savings account to pay for a shopping splurge instead of accumulating more calorie debt. The temporary pleasure was gone, leaving remorse to be sucked into the vacuum it created in my conscience. The muffins had tasted good going down, the apple chunks juicy yet crispy, the cinnamon and Splenda sweet and delicious. But now I didn't feel so good. I thought I might throw up, from binging or from self-disgust, I wasn't sure.

It was as if a child had grabbed my hand and was using it to smack my face repeatedly while chanting, "Why are you hitting yourself? Why are you hitting yourself?" I should just get over it already. I was doing so well the other 95 percent of the time. Focusing on the 5 percent that I screwed up was like getting upset that I didn't have a perfect SAT score. I couldn't change the past, and I didn't live in the future. I could control only the here and now. It sounded good in theory. Now if I could only get myself to live this Zen philosophy.

I wasn't a 100 percent perfect dieter. No one was. If I fell out of bed, I wouldn't call myself a failure at sleeping. I'd get up and make a note to sleep toward the middle of the bed. My mother liked to say I was a work in progress. It was hard to progress if you were always perfect.

It was also hard to progress if you were in a weight plateau. I hated the word plateau. It was hard to spell. Didn't the French fear a vowel shortage? My weight loss had followed a boom and bust cycle in the past. I frequently lost a lot of weight the week of my period and then held steady for the next three weeks. Then I'd descend again around the next time of the month. Now I was just stalled.

I'd hit a couple of plateaus before, once in the 280s and again in the 260s. Now I'd built another camp in the 220s. Even when I wasn't inhaling muffins like oxygen, the number wouldn't budge. It was frustrating because I was still exercising and eating the same way as when I'd been losing weight, but I wasn't getting the same results.

There were weigh-in tricks I could have pulled. I was always sure to pee before I weighed myself in the mornings. Some people avoided sodium the night before a weigh-in so they wouldn't be bloated. Others skipped dinner all together. I took off my watch once and lost about 2 ounces. I considered weighing in naked, an option I hadn't had at the house. The scale had been kept in the front closet because there was no space on the bathroom floor. Getting a new low number on the scale was like getting a new high score on a video game, but I wasn't going to risk running into my brother naked in the hallway to get it. In the western corner of Niger obesity was considered attractive and women actually put on scarves or hats before weighing themselves.[1] I found this impossible to imagine.

My blog had started to develop a small following and everyone online gave me advice about my plateau, even though I couldn't recall asking for any. I hadn't gotten this much unsolicited advice since the last time I'd had the hiccups. I was told by my blog readers to cut carbs, reduce my fat intake, join Weight Watchers, eat a tablespoon of canola oil during lunch to reset my hunger levels, and become a vegetarian. Had I considered yoga? One person asked if I'd read about the intuitive eating philosophy, which said you should eat what you wanted to, but only when you were hungry. If I'd been able to do that to begin with, I would never have gotten so fat.

Another person suggested that I'd reached my set point. This was a theory that everyone had a natural weight his or her body wanted to stabilize at.[2] If I had a set point, why had my body let me get so fat to begin with? Some people said the set point could be raised if you gained weight, but not as easily lowered when you lost weight. The set-point theory didn't make much sense when applied to my personal weight history. I doubted I had ever been calibrated to 372 pounds because I had lost about 150 pounds without ever feeling hungry or deprived. The set-point theory would have been nice if it functioned like an emergency shutoff valve that stopped me from getting fatter than a certain weight, but it didn't seem to work like that for me. There were always new scientific theories explaining how the complex organic machine that was my body functioned. I had no idea which ones were true or not.

I wasn't going to give up because of small bouts of resistance. Some of my readers sounded as if they were trying to let me down easy and prevent my heart from breaking if I never got to goal. It was like I was playing *Who Wants to Be a Millionaire?* and they wanted me to leave with the $250,000 instead of trying for a million.

I knew what I was willing to do to manage my weight and how much time I was willing to put into it. I was willing to challenge myself. I was willing to walk farther and faster. I was willing to cut back on food now that I was thinner and didn't need as many calories to keep my heart beating and lungs breathing. I wouldn't be happy until I knew I'd pushed myself as far as I was willing to go. I hadn't reached that point yet.

The plateau might have been good exercise for my mind. It built up my ability to persist through times of failure.[3] I had read that scientists believed persistence was governed by a circuit in the brain. Some people naturally had higher levels of persistence than others. Their brains told them to keep trying through the hard times because there was a reward at the end that would stimulate their pleasure centers when they succeeded. Fortunately, even if you started out with a low level of persistence, you could be trained to have more if you were not rewarded every time you accomplished a task. My brain was like an old lady in a casino who kept feeding coins into the slots because she knew the next one would bury her up to her granny panties in coins. When I did eventually start losing weight again, I was training myself that if I kept trying, the rewards would come. It also meant I should take a vacation in Vegas. The casinos obviously had lots to teach me.

I eventually burst through my plateau, if only by force of habit. I was used to exercising and eating healthily, so I just kept doing that. It had become my new default setting. My weight loss also kept slowing down the closer I got to my goal weight. My body was smaller, so I wasn't burning as many calories a day. Bodies were highly adaptable. If you pushed them one way, they pushed back in the opposite direction. If I didn't drink much water, my body would start retaining it. If I ran a lot, my body became more efficient at running. It could accomplish the task at a lower energy cost, like a grocery shopper on triple-coupon day. Losing weight was like trying to pass another car on the highway, only to have it speed up every time I made a move in the left lane. The secret wasn't to pass the car at full throttle but to zigzag and confuse it until I could slip by. I needed to mix up my exercise routine and vary what I ate to keep my body from thinking it needed to store fat. My body didn't care how good my butt looked in jeans. It cared about not dying. If I were living in a time when food was scarce, I would outlive all those people who were naturally skinny and couldn't keep their fat cells full after eating a bucket of chicken wings.

I decided to set early August of the next year as D-day. I wouldn't be storming the beaches of Normandy, although that would be great cardio. No, this was the date my older brother had set for his wedding. I'd weigh 160 pounds or else . . . I'd have to buy a bigger dress.

No matter how long I'd been at this, I noticed that I always seemed to be a year away from my goal. The previous fall I'd celebrated my birthday by determining that at my current rate of loss I'd be at goal in a year. Many months later I was still a year away from goal. What strange twisting of space-time was this? It made me think of Zeno's Paradox: To get from point A to point B you must first travel halfway there. Once you got halfway there you had to then travel halfway between the remaining distance. Then you had to travel halfway again. You had to continue doing this infinitely, which begged the question, "How the hell did we actually manage to go anywhere at all?" I didn't know.

I did know that we managed to get from point A to point B. I could get to goal too, but I would have to struggle through the dieting trifecta of doom first: Halloween, Thanksgiving, and Christmas. During this time I had to pass candy displays built in the middle of the grocery store, monuments of tribute to a religion I no longer practiced. The landscape for those months consisted of fields of candy corn, a sky full of pumpkin pies, and a sea of eggnog with creamy foam breakers. The abundance of feast holidays during the winter months might have heralded from the need to eat more when it was colder. Or people just loved an excuse to eat like pigs.

Thanksgiving and Christmas were supposed to be times to celebrate family and life, but it was also time to pay tribute to my gastric system. When I heard the magic clinking of green and red M&M's being poured into a glass bowl, I still came skittering around the corner like my cat when he heard kibble bouncing into his bowl. Pavlov might have had something to say about that, but I wouldn't have heard him over the crunching in my mouth.

When I snuck a peek at the scale two days after Christmas to weigh the damage I'd done with chocolate-covered cherries and candy canes, I discovered I'd lost two pounds. Perhaps all the chocolate acted as a laxative? I couldn't explain it. After my Christmas bender, I confessed my sins on the blog, like a good old-fashioned Catholic. Bless me, Father, for I have binged. I had been to a Catholic confession only once before I'd stopped going to church, but I spilled my eating sins online much more frequently, waiting for forgiveness from my readers. If only my body would have granted me indulgences like the church used to. For a small fee I could have gotten my dieting sins erased.

The holidays were different these days because I *did* feel guilty. In previous years I could eat half a pumpkin pie and a tub of whipped cream on Thanksgiving and feel fine about it. I had no idea how many calories it had or how badly it would affect my body. Now I was enlightened, thrown out of the Garden of Eden with only an apple to munch on.

As I went through life, I acquired and lost certain filters. The things happening in my life, be it my job or losing weight, shaped the way I looked at the world. When I worked at a copy store for a year designing resumes and business cards, I not only got a regular paycheck but also developed the "Compulsively Identify Fonts" filter. Customers frequently requested that we re-create an item exactly, so I had to learn to identify fonts. Within a week of starting, I nearly collided with a car on the expressway because I couldn't keep my eyes off a billboard with an unidentifiable sans serif font. I saw the musical *Ragtime* and spent thirty seconds of the show distracted by a banner on stage, trying to determine if it used Bodoni Poster or Britannic Bold. I couldn't watch television without randomly yelling out font names used in commercials, seeing glares not from light bouncing off the TV screen but from my family. When my job was eventually eliminated and we were all laid off, I was grateful because I finally stopped randomly yelling the names of dead font designers like a Tourette's sufferer.

Since I started losing weight, I had acquired the "You're Actually Going to Eat That Crap?" filter. At my extended family's Christmas Eve dinner it was kicked into overdrive at the sight of deep-fried chicken set next to potato salad slathered in mayonnaise, which was low fat only in comparison to a bathtub full of chicken fat. This filter made me a judgmental asshole, but I at least had the sense to be a silent judgmental asshole. I couldn't turn off the filter even if I wanted to. Two years ago a pepperoni pizza made me think *Yum!* and now it made me think *Is that cheese low fat?*

Unlike the font filter, this was a good filter to have. It kept me from gaining weight. But if I were to ignore it for too long, it would probably have faded away just like my other filters. It also made me painfully aware of how poorly my fellow citizens ate. I'd never realized this when I was one of them.

Social eating was the most frequent trigger for a slipup. When I was in my own kitchen, the worst thing I could do, other than cut a finger off, was to eat an entire bowl of sugar-free, fat-free pudding. Out in the real world, the gun was loaded, the safety was off, and I was a dollar menu away from shooting myself in my pinky toe. I wanted to be part of the group and celebrate birthdays and anniversaries at restaurants, but it was difficult to do that without overeating. Sometimes I wished I were an alcoholic so I'd have a good excuse not to go out drinking.

I found myself pondering how many calories were in a single M&M. I didn't know because I'd never eaten only one M&M, unless I unearthed it in the sofa cushions while searching for the remote control. Surely stale M&M's lost calories with age, like the half-life of radioactive materials. After doing some division, I determined that there are 3.4 calories in a milk chocolate M&M. I looked it up after attending a baby shower for a woman (and baby) I didn't even know, because it had been a better question to ponder at the time than "If I faked a folding-chair malfunction to break my arm, would they let me leave for the hospital immediately or make me wait fifteen minutes for an ambulance?"

As with any social event, I had to face "The Trial of the Buffet Table." The candy-corn cups and vanilla cake and sherbet were easily avoided because I'd eaten two hours beforehand. Vanilla wasn't even in the same league of dieting temptations as chocolate. Each guest also received a foam flower centerpiece in a miniature flowerpot containing a bag of M&Ms. Earlier in the year I had read a study that showed people were more likely to eat candy if it were put within easy reach.[4] You didn't have to be a researcher at the University of Illinois at Urbana-Champaign to know that! I'd figured it out by the third handful.

I lasted an hour before I started digging into my flowerpot, just a couple at first and then some more until I'd eventually eaten thirty candies out of boredom. At least I'd squashed my ability to scream by filling my mouth with chocolate. Otherwise I would have yelled, "Why must the baby have two dozen blankets?! Is she going to be sleeping in the freezer?"

At least I didn't face pressures like this at work. My company had three employees including me. There were no birthday parties with cupcakes, no boxes of donuts lying in the lobby, no Christmas parties where I'd have to trip the waiter serving hors d'oeuvres to prevent myself from pigging out. It was just me, the microwave, and my Lean Cuisines. Once or twice my boss suggested ordering pizza and I told him, "No thanks." I didn't have health insurance, but the low-pressure eating environment was doing wonders for my health.

My health had been doing wonders for my family's health too. Several months after my mother sold the house and we had all moved to our own apartments, she called me. "Hey," I said, recognizing her familiar voice. I put down my fork. I was eating dinner way too fast like I always did. I needed to slow down and enjoy the food, but I still ate as if I were trying to win a hotdog-eating contest.

"Hi," she replied warmly. "I was just calling to thank you."

"Oh, for what?"

"For keeping all that junk food out of the house," she said. "I've been kind of bad lately, eating a lot of ice cream. My blood sugar has gone up." My mother was not diabetic but her mother had been, and the doctor was being particularly rigorous in preventing Mom from following in her footsteps. She checked her blood sugar frequently and went in for quarterly checkups. "I just wanted to thank you for keeping us eating healthy."

"You're welcome," I said, smiling a little, surprised by her gratitude. It was funny how people would do things for others that they wouldn't do for themselves. "I guess healthy eating and weight loss are contagious. I need to infect you again."

"That would be good," she said. "Oh, do you have the recipe for the turkey meat loaf?"

CHAPTER 13

My Online Waistline

It was just December 2006 that I had been waiting on a secret phone call from my contact in Japan. I didn't want my mother to know, so I had set my cell phone to vibrate and tucked it into my pocket, pretending to be interested in Bruce Willis's climbing an elevator shaft in the festive Christmas movie, *Die Hard*.

This, of course, had to do with the blog.

If I let my mother know about the call, I'd have to reveal my secret identity as PastaQueen, weight-loss blogger extraordinaire and inventor of the rotating progress photos. I wasn't ready to reveal my dual life just yet. This was the closest I'd ever felt to being a superhero.

I don't remember why I started the blog. I guess I wanted to understand myself and to be understood by others. I suspect it was partly because I had a lot of fat issues that I needed to work out. Most of my life had been spent trying *not* to think about my fat, part of my unsuccessful life philosophy that if you ignored something it would go away. Posting my thoughts online put an end to that. The blog wasn't a food diary or an exercise log. I barely cared what I'd eaten last week, so I doubted anyone else would. Instead it was a place where I thought about my fat and all the baggage that came with it. If I thought about my problems, I started to understand them, and then I could work to overcome them. I wrote entries in my head while walking the endless loop of the treadmill, thinking and losing weight at the same time.

Fame whoring was probably involved too. I'd always enjoyed writing and knew some writers had carved out their own niches in cyberspace. If only a thousand people watched a TV show, it would be a flop. But if a thousand people visited your blog every day, it would be considered a mild success. It was a web "site" after all, a place to stake my ground and build something new.

I wasn't too eager to pimp my wares at first. I didn't tell anyone, online or offline, about the blog until nine months and a hundred pounds into my weight loss. I didn't know if I were going to be a success story. I wasn't eager to have my family and friends share in the disappointment if my "after" photo ended up looking just like my "before" photo, with different lighting and one more grease stain on my blouse. I felt vulnerable. I didn't want anyone reading unless she'd stumbled upon the site while searching for an industrial weight scale.

I performed similar searches myself, looking for blogs written by people with butts as big as my own. Men dominated many arenas online, but women ruled the fat blogs. Women certainly have more to gain by losing weight since they are judged more on their looks than men. I didn't know too many men who wouldn't go outside without their mascara. I'd also learned obese people were paid less than their thin counterparts, and that the differential was the largest for fat, white women.[1] Guess who was writing most of these blogs?

I decided to leave a comment on one of the sites. I entered my name and email address into the form and then paused. The cursor blinked in a white text box next to the "website" field. If I entered my site's address, anyone who read my comment could click on the link and read my blog. I entered my web address but then hammered the backspace button as if I were sending out Morse code. Then I stopped.

I entered my web address again and clicked "Submit."

I left comments on other blogs during the next couple of weeks. After that, I noticed ads for diet programs, plus-size retailers, and weight-loss surgery popping up repeatedly when I was browsing, even on sites that had nothing to do with obesity. Somehow my computer knew that I was fat. I could only assume it had been gossiping about me with other computers behind my back. If I removed some of its memory as punishment, would it forget the circumference of my thighs?

I came home from work a few days later, checked my email, and found a notification in my inbox. Someone had left a comment on *my* blog. I had gotten a couple of comments before. One was from a woman who was on a "three dat diet" and said "Ineed help." The only help I wanted to give her involved whacking a dictionary against her head. Maybe if I swung it hard enough, the proper rules of spelling would be transferred from the pages into her head? The other comment was from a woman who had confused me for the thousand-pound man I had written about.

The latest comment was from Mark, my Japanese contact, who had visited my blog after I left a comment on his. Several months later Mark asked me to post some entries on his site while he was away during the holidays. This was the source of my Christmas subterfuge. A couple of weeks later more people started visiting my virtual open house after another blogger wrote an entry about how much she liked my rotating progress photos. I had created interactive images that let users spin me around like clay on a pottery wheel, checking out the size of my ass from eight different angles. Someone said it was like dancing with me. Soon my dance card got pretty full.

My blog didn't become popular overnight, but through the months more and more visitors started showing up on my site statistics page. I watched these statistics more closely than I will ever admit, and I was excited when I saw that a new site had linked to me or that my monthly page views had increased. It was a popularity contest in which the fat girl was actually winning.

I spent a weekend redesigning the look of the site, upgrading from the default template I'd been using. If people were dropping by, I felt obligated to clean up the place. I'd named my blog "Half of Me" because I needed to lose half my body weight. Actually, I needed to lose four-sevenths of me, but that wasn't as catchy. I took the progress photo of myself at my fattest, staring glumly at the camera, and split it down the middle, lopping off my head for good measure. I placed it in the left column, looming huge on the screen, though still not as large as I was in real life.

It was scary. My progress photos were much smaller and seques-tered away on their own page, but this would be the first image people would see when they visited the site. It was shocking and unattract-ive. The truth often was. I was keeping my blog clandestine from the real world, yet my obesity was obvious to anyone with a functioning retina. It was a secret I kept hidden in a glass box, locked away but visible to all.

When I copied and pasted that photo into my site design, I felt as if I'd taken the eraser tool and begun to wipe away some of my shame. It was important to post photos that were real. Telling someone I was fat frequently sounded like a judgment of my character, as if it were something to be ashamed of. When I posted the pictures and started talking about my weight openly, I started to see weight simply as a description of myself, not a judgment of my character. I didn't have to pretend to be the best Photoshopped version of myself. I didn't have to give myself perfect skin with the diffuse glow filter or eliminate my double chin with the clone stamp. I could just be myself, fat rolls and all.

Now that I wasn't the only one watching my weight, I felt more responsibility to keep going. I posted my poundage every Saturday to track my progress. I would have hesitated if one of my coworkers asked me how much I weighed. I hadn't even told my family what my highest weight was until I'd lost a hundred pounds of it, yet I had no problem posting that integer online for millions of people to see. I figured my friends and family were unlikely to find the blog, and I didn't particularly care what a bunch of strangers thought about a headless fat girl from Indiana.

I started to get some regular readers who told me my journey was a "thinspiration" and it wouldn't be long before I was in "one-derland," the place where my weight would begin with the digit one. We were all on a weight-loss journey, but I don't know where we were supposed to be going. Maybe we'd hit the all-you-can-eat buffet when we got there and start all over again? Wherever it was, the thought of having to post a gain for more than two weeks in a row kept my foot off the brake. Private failure would have been tolerable. Public failure was not an option. I was convinced that if I gave up, they'd knock down my door with a twenty-pound dumbbell and chain me to the treadmill with a yoga strap until I promised to reach goal.

I was a somewhat cynical person, preferring chicken soup for my stomach, not for my soul, but I found myself becoming more and more of a shmoopy cheerleader. All my newfound wisdom kept spilling out of my head to be mopped up in the blog. My readers made me feel so good. They were happy for me when I lost weight and reassured me during the long plateaus (when they weren't annoying me with unsolicited advice). We were all fighting fat and we formed bonds like any war buddies. One woman emailed to tell me she had prayed for me to lose weight during my latest plateau. I didn't know whether to be flattered or to get a post office box for my public domain listing.

Before the blog, I wouldn't have gone out of my way to meet a fiftysomething woman in the middle of nowhere who read blogs while knitting perched on a stability ball. But now I knew people in Australia and Scotland and even some place called Nebraska. As the months went by, people lost jobs and found new ones, got married or broke up. They ran marathons. Some even created whole new people. The residents of the blogosphere were rather cool, though the word "blogosphere" brought humorous images to my mind. I imagined us moving into the old Biosphere 2 project in the desert, a complex of geodesic domes where we could grow our own soy products.

It was always disturbing when a blogger went missing. There was one woman whose entries about how our lives were shaped by our size made me ponder my perspective on the world in whole new ways. She vanished in the spring. There was a woman who would analyze the emotional and nutritional reasons behind overeating in amazing detail. She evaporated in the middle of summer. The time between their posts kept getting longer and longer or they would only pop in to write, "Gee whiz! I sure haven't posted lately, have I?" When they disappeared completely it was probably not because their laptops had been stolen. It usually meant only one thing.

They'd started gaining weight.

That or they were dead, a serious possibility for the morbidly obese.

Whenever I started gaining weight, I went out less and less. I avoided friends from high school or college who'd known me when I was thinner. It made sense that bloggers would do the same thing online. Ironically, this was the time they needed to keep blogging the most, but they were probably ashamed of the bruises they got from falling off the wagon. Sometimes I thought the wagon must have a maximum safe-weight capacity, which was why people kept getting pushed off. It wasn't helping that they were avoiding the people who could relate to them most. My readers were a constant source of support and motivation. When I read their comments, I chose to believe most of the two-dimensional comments on my screen were attached to three-dimensional people who cared about me.

Had the missing completely given up hope? If you were blogging, you were thinking about your goal. If you stopped thinking about your goal, you would stop losing weight too. There was a girl who commented on my blog for several weeks, inspired by my progress and gung-ho to do the same. I was really rooting for her, and then she vanished. When she deleted her blog, I felt like I'd witnessed someone commit online suicide. I never did find out what happened to her.

I'd been there too, when nothing seemed to work, and I thought I'd be fat for the rest of my life. I wanted to hide away from the world and live under my bedspread in a blanket fort and train the bedbugs to perform tricks in a circus. But I knew that wasn't the answer and not just because the bedbugs would unionize and cause labor problems.

I wanted to find all the missing bloggers and let them know that someone had noticed they were gone. Many of them remain missing, the reason for their absence still unknown. Only their blog archives remain standing like lost Mayan civilizations, the only proof of their creators' previous existence.

Fat chicks weren't the only ones interested in the blog. I got an email from a company requesting that I test its soda-making machine. I declined despite my curiosity. The company contacted me right before I was moving, and I didn't want to carry a soda machine up the stairs in addition to my hundreds of pounds of books. I wrote a negative review for a yoga DVD and months later the instructor's publishing company offered me a free copy of her new book to review anyway. I wondered if anyone had bothered reading my post. A TV show's producer wrote to me about possibly appearing on a new talk show to discuss how my relationships had changed since losing weight. I turned the offer down.

People didn't just want to send me weird crap to review. I offhandedly mentioned that my right hand got cold at work because it was on a computer mouse all day, far away from my body heat. The next week I came home to find a brown paper package on my welcome mat with a pair of knitted wrist-warmers sent by a reader. I should have gone the Rumpelstiltskin route and inquired what she could do with straw. Another woman sent me a book I'd mentioned I'd wanted but didn't have the money to buy.

I started playing a sweepstakes in which every lid on my yogurt cups contained an entry code. One of my readers started sending me her contest numbers too. After consuming about sixty cups of yogurt and 3,600 calories from an unknown number of live bacteria cultures, I finally won a gift certificate with one of her codes. Gambling wasn't just a painful addiction that could lead to financial distress and emotional turmoil. It could also lead you to eat lots of dairy.

The more weight I lost, the more people were impressed. It was no big deal when I lost a pound or two a week, but when I repeated that process for months on end, people were awed. Visitors were now seeing almost two years of progress at once, like a time-lapse photo. Some people started reading all my archives in a day, as if they'd died and my life had passed before their eyes instead of their own.

I was an inspiration. I had been told so 876 times. I got questions about what I was eating, what exercise DVDs I used, and what diet I was on. When had *I* become a weight-loss guru? Didn't you have to at least drop out of medical school before you pretended to be a health expert?

I felt like a sideshow preacher being asked to heal the sick with her magic hands. I suppose anyone who reads enough about a subject can become an expert. I was certainly doing something right, but I wasn't sure if I even knew what it was. It was like asking a bird what the four principles of flight were.

But I loved it. I had found two things I was good at—losing weight and writing—and I was getting praise for them both. I wanted more web traffic, and I wanted to lose more weight. I wanted to get to goal and host a celebration party inside of my fat pants.

I was helping people too, of course. I wasn't a *completely* self-centered blog whore, even though blogging about my weight was by definition rather self-centered. It was important for people to know someone was out there succeeding. My blog wasn't a guarantee that they could succeed, but it showed that losing the weight was possible. There was great power in showing people possibilities.

I was also a real person who would email them back. I wasn't an infomercial where you couldn't be sure if the before and after pictures featured different actresses and digital effects. Just as I had been motivated to lose weight because my brother had, people said they'd started attempting to lose weight because of my blog. They tried Pilates because I'd mentioned I'd liked it. Reading the details of my loss week by week made the goal seem more achievable to people than if they'd just seen the beginning and end results. It had a thrilling live element too. You never knew what would happen next week. Would PastaQueen get to goal? Or would she crash and burn in a red hot blaze of chili cheese dogs?

One day I checked my email and received this comment:

> *I have spent the last two weeks in my office reading your*
> *blog (while no one was looking) and I have finally gotten to a*

point where I just don't feel like I want to die anymore. I feel like
there is hope. Thank you. SO MUCH. I have something to look
forward to in my life. I can do this.

Wow. I stared at the screen and read the comment again. Damn. I'd just wanted to stop shopping in the plus-size section and now someone had told me I'd saved her life.

Holy crap, I was a role model.

Was I worthy of being a role model? I just wanted to reduce the size of my ass. As a bonus, the blog was a stamp of validation on the parking garage ticket of my life. It was a great change from the days when I never thought I'd do anything meaningful with my life and had kept the television company all day. Weight loss had become my big project. I'd never known how to make my life better, but I had been able to do it by writing my blog and reshaping my body and my mind. Now I was being treated like a glaring beacon of hope. I didn't know what to think of that.

When I started losing weight, the blog was the only place I let my ideas and feelings about my weight be known. God forbid I actually talk to friends and family about my fatness. I had always felt the most like myself in my writing. I could be bold and witty on the page or the computer screen, but in real life I was still the shy girl hiding behind a mess of curls. I often wished I was as brave as my blog. As I wrote more frequently, thought more about who I was, and engaged in positive self-talk with other women in the blogosphere, I found myself believing I *could* be the same funny, confident girl in the three-dimensional world as I was in the world of modems and fiber-optic cables.

Many people consider the online community to be fake or substandard to day-to-day human interactions, but the confidence I found in this "fake" universe started to slowly bleed into my real life.

I started making small talk with strangers more easily, in elevators or theater halls. At a family reunion I actually talked to my family. I got the guts to sign up for a kickboxing class because other bloggers did aerobics. The closest I'd come to kickboxing previously was the time I stubbed my toe on a cardboard box of books during my move.

I hoped these people were fans of my writing. If they were just fans of my weight loss, that would be a little weird. Some visitors did seem more interested in my weekly weigh-ins than I was. After I posted a gain they would console me and tell me it was only a temporary setback. I already knew this. It was practically impossible to lose weight every single week. There was no reason to get hysterical about it. I felt like they were swarming me with full medical attention over a small paper cut. Some seemed to be living vicariously through my own weight loss. One visitor said she had to remind herself that just because I was losing weight didn't mean she was.

It was a lot more fun celebrating major milestones with all my readers. What use was good news if you didn't have someone to share it with? Eventually I started to weigh less than some of the bloggers I'd been reading. I hoped they didn't hate me. I'd never been fond of the upstart freshman flautist, who practiced hard every night and eventually stole my chair junior year of band.

One of my readers compared my slimmer pictures to Jennifer Connelly or Katie Holmes. This was much more flattering than the last time I'd been compared to a celebrity. I'd submitted my picture to an online tool that calculated which famous person you most looked like and had been told I resembled Brendan Fraser.

The visitors were also a living encyclopedia of weight-loss information. When I wanted to start weight lifting, they were quick to recommend DVDs. When I proclaimed my new love of oatmeal, they posted links to tasty recipes. If anyone ever overstepped the bounds of the blogger/reader relationship by telling me to move back in with my mother or suggesting I go to therapy, there was always the "Delete Comment" button.

Surprisingly, I received very few hateful comments. I had thought my big, fat photos would be a big, fat target. When I did get nasty responses they were almost always misspelled and lacked proper capitalization, making them easy to rationalize away; I didn't understand why people would think I would respect their opinion if they couldn't be bothered to hit the shift key. Using improper capitalization and poor spelling when you commented on a blog for the first time was like meeting someone while you weren't wearing any pants. It didn't make a good impression.

In January my site traffic doubled. Weight-loss resolutions were great for my page views. I tried to post at least three to four times a week so they'd keep coming back, which was difficult to manage while working full time and sticking to an exercise schedule. One Monday morning I realized I hadn't posted anything since Thursday and whipped up an entry quickly before I went to work. I read through it once for grammatical errors, posted it, grabbed a peach, and walked out the door.

By the time I got to work and checked my email, I realized why writers needed editors. My entry had accidentally implied that people who needed to lose only thirty pounds were not as serious about weight loss as people who had to lose more than one hundred pounds. This wasn't what I had intended to say at all; I had just been sloppy choosing my words. I had meant to say that I'd always viewed this as a long-term project because I had so much weight to drop, but I phrased it in a way that could be read as disrespectful to people who hadn't weighed nearly four hundred pounds.

I started to get some angry comments. That wasn't right. The Internet was supposed to love me. I was an inspiration. They'd told me so. They wanted to hoist me up in my ergonomic desk chair and parade me through the streets as I threw sugar-free candies to the crowds.

Now the Internet *hated* me. My parade had turned into a lynch mob.

I had sometimes been scared to post entries about personal topics or controversial ideas, but I did it anyway because words weren't made for cowards. Usually I was rewarded with an "I totally agree" or a "Hell, yeah!" While I knew it shouldn't matter if anyone agreed with me, it totally did. It became easier and easier to speak up when I knew people liked what I was saying. Sometimes there was a polite dissent, which usually led to interesting conversations. Now people were more pissed than I'd ever seen them before.

I tried to explain my error in the comments section. Some regular readers beat me to it and jumped to my defense. I could smell the gas leak filling the room with combustible materials. I needed to turn off the valve before someone lit a spark and my blog exploded. I disabled comments on the entry. I was scared to check my email for a day afterward. Every time my computer dinged with a new message, I'd take a deep breath as I clicked on my inbox, hoping someone hadn't taken time to write me a nasty email. To my surprise no one bothered to send me hate mail. Hmmm. It was possible I was not as important as I thought I was.

In the scheme of things, it was only a minor tiff. When I'd first started blogging, a mommy blogger had written a post implying that women who gained weight after they got married were guilty of false advertising to their husbands. That's not exactly what she wrote, but that's what people heard and that's all that mattered. The Internet eviscerated her. They dragged her into the public square, plucked the keys off their keyboards, and stoned her to death with F11 buttons. Then they strung her up with their mouse cords to hang. I didn't agree with everything she had said, but no one deserved that. I had cringed when reading their comments and it wasn't even my blog. I imagined she must have been curled under her desk rocking back and forth in the fetal position and mumbling to herself, "It's just a blog. It's just a blog."

Luckily for me, no one would even remember my stupid blog blowout a month later. The Internet was capricious. I'd put a lot of my self-worth into the popularity of my blog, but my readers could turn on me unexpectedly. It was a conditional love. There were many people I'd met through the blog whom I considered true friends, but most of my readers were strangers. They might feel as if they knew me because they'd read my blog, but I had no idea who most of them were. They were usually very nice, but it might be in my best interest not to let my self-esteem get too wrapped up in what they thought of me. How many of them would still love me if I gained back a hundred pounds? It might make me more sympathetic and real, but people loved a good success story.

And I desperately wanted to be a success story. So many people gained back the weight. They might keep it off for a year or two or three, but a study had recently been released saying dieting didn't work and that most people gained all the weight back within five years.[2] The study didn't bother me too much because it defined dieting as "severely restricting one's calorie intake to lose weight," which I wasn't doing. I would have sucked at that anyway. I'd recently forgotten to bring my cheese sticks to work again and had sat at my desk letting the hunger gnaw away instead of going to the vending machine. By the time I got home I almost ate the plastic wrapper with the cheese because I was so hungry. I just couldn't do the starvation thing. The press release for the study also said, "Eating in moderation is a good idea for everybody, and so is regular exercise," which *was* what I was doing. So if I eventually failed it wasn't going to be because diets didn't work. I wasn't on a diet.

I still gained weight sometimes, and I made myself report it online as part of my promised weekly weigh-in. There were some weeks I seriously considered lying. Who would know? They couldn't come to my house and weigh me. They didn't demand photographs of my feet on the scale. I could fudge a pound or two and no one would know.

I just couldn't do it, though. These people took comfort in knowing someone had lost so much weight. I couldn't pretend it was a piece of cake, even if I weren't eating much cake. Weight loss could be so hard. It was important for them to know that you could win the war and still lose some battles. My blog kept me from making excuses. I had to face that number every week no matter what.

I edited the template and rebuilt my site to reflect the new larger number on the scale, and I immediately felt depressed. I might have just been bored or I might not have had enough caffeine, or it could have been premenstrual hormones. Whatever. I ravaged my kitchen like the Vikings pillaging a village and immediately regretted it. I didn't want to let these people down. If I failed, it was as though we all failed. It was like having your favorite baseball team lose the World Series, which was ridiculous and self-important of me to think. I may have been calling myself PastaQueen, but I wasn't queen of the weight-loss bloggers. If my site disappeared there would always be women to take my place. But I still wanted to prove it was possible to lose lots of weight and keep it off. I had so much sympathy for people who did regain the weight. I understood how it could happen, but I did not want to join the I-regained-one-hundred-pounds club. It could save its membership card and keep me off the club's mailing list.

I watched some TV. No one expected me to be perfect, except me. I loved so many things about the blogging community, but I didn't owe it anything. The only pressure was the pressure I put on myself. But on days like this I felt like I was slipping just a bit, as if I had twisted my ankle and was waving my arms to avoid falling face first, splat, onto the gravel path. I hadn't fallen over yet, but it could happen and I had to keep waving my arms or gravity would have its way with me.

It made me wonder, *who was that girl on the blog who was so optimistic and motivated and inspiring?* I did not feel like her today. She was out for a run and I hoped she'd return to my body tomorrow. I should read my blog and take my own damned advice instead of sitting around moping.

I had no desire to leave my apartment, but I went for a walk. There used to be a time in my life when I could eat half the cupboards' contents and barely feel a smidge of guilt, but those days were over. This was sad in some ways, but mostly not. Even after I took my walk, I wouldn't burn off all the calories I'd eaten, but at least I'd burn some of them. I hoped the activity would make me feel peppier too. I hadn't gotten half a mile down the trail before I started thinking, "You could just turn around now and go home. You don't have to do this." But I knew there was no turning back. If I turned back, I was screwed. Going back was not an option. If I looked back, I'd turn into a pillar of salt and somebody's dog would lick me up and poop me out.

Every step of that first mile was drudgery and I hated it, but by the second mile I started to feel a bit better, and by the third mile I was happy to be out there in the world, and by the fourth mile I was proud to be a person who could walk four miles at all. Especially when a one-armed man ran by me and I thought, *At least you can do something about your weight. That guy's never going to grow back his arm.*

I would probably still gain weight today. And I was never going to like that. But I would do my best tomorrow and the day after that and the day after that and hope that I would lose weight on more days than I gained weight. And I could do this whether I had a blog or not. Onward I would go because backward was not an option.

Then my mom found the blog.

I was sitting on the plush brown couch in her apartment when she told me. We'd just finished a turkey dinner, though a meal with chicken would have been more reflective of my attitude about her discovery.

"By the way," she said apropos of nothing from the vinyl recliner. "I found your blog."

I wanted to curl up in the fetal position, which I could physically do now. I always knew that my relatives could find the blog accidentally, but I wasn't sending out engraved invitations with the web address on them, either. I never thought my mom would crash my online party. That's what I got for teaching her how to use Google. Now my family would know exactly who I was. This was the scariest thing about emblogessment. They would see me as I was around my online friends, which was not always the same way I was around my family. Yes, my mother had cared for me and fed me (obviously) and loved me, but we never know everything about those we love. I'd said things on my blog I'd never said to anyone. Losing weight had provided an opportunity for growth, a way for me to find out who I was, and most of that was chronicled on the blog. I'd put all my vulnerable, fleshy bits out there for everyone to see, and that came with the risk of getting poked with a stick.

"Oh," I mumbled through the hands covering my face. "What did you think of it?"

"It's really great!" she said. "Your rotating progress photos are fun."

Thank God she didn't mention the muffins I'd baked in the shape of vaginas. I'd experimented in healthy erotic baking to celebrate my friend's performance in *The Vagina Monologues*.

I sped home that night and vowed to read all my archives. I had been too scared to read my two years' worth of entries, but this event required instant mom-proofing. The thought of reading my blog in its entirety induced enough anxiety, fear, and paranoia that I started wishing for a Xanax and a chaser of rum. I couldn't remember what I'd written. It would be like looking at old yearbook photos. What if I discovered I'd had a mullet? I couldn't remember how revealing I'd been when I had assumed no one was reading. It was a lot easier to dance like no one was watching when no one was in the room with a camera phone.

I booted up my computer, surfed to my site, and made a sharp right turn onto memory lane. Suddenly I was a fat girl again, thighs rubbing together as I walked down the sidewalk, panting and out of breath. Sadness and hopelessness littered the street like roadkill and potholes. I'd forgotten how unhappy I'd been, wondering if I'd ever find a way off this dilapidated road. But as I continued my trip, the pavement started to get smoother, and the construction project started to show progress. Flowers were blooming in the center of the parkway, and the all-you-can-eat restaurants started to disappear. The road ahead seemed to lead somewhere instead of stopping at a dead end.

I'd finally figured it out, without the help of a cartographer. This was the journey we were all on. I'd just never realized how far I'd come. Good thing I'd left a map.

CHAPTER 14

Acquired Tastes

I wanted to eat the star fruit because it was cute.

I bought most of my fruits at the grocery store based on looks. I didn't know if that thin layer of wax on an apple's skin made it taste better, but it sure did make it look shiny. I always reached for the apples with the deep, red coloring over the ones with spots or discolorations. If apples were people, I was a bigoted looksist. The star fruit was a light yellow-green, kind of waxy, and the size of a miniature football. When I picked it up and stared down its end, it looked like a five-pointed star.

I ripped a plastic bag off the dispenser, bagged the star fruit, and gently placed it in my cart. When I got home, I eagerly grabbed my cutting board and cut off several slices of the fruit. They were shaped like delightful little stars. They reminded me of an art project in grade school in which we cut a star shape into the bottom of a potato and used it as a stamp. I bit into the green star and savored the slightly crunchy, lime-like taste. This wasn't bad. It was kind of expensive to buy on a regular basis, but the adorable shape made the eating experience so much fun.

When I returned to the grocery store a week later it didn't have any star fruit in stock. As I looked around, I realized there was a lot of fruit that I usually ignored. There were vegetables I still didn't know the names of. I had never bought any of these items because . . . I had no good reason. I typically shopped for food off a list or grabbed items I was familiar with. I tuned out any extraneous data the way I ignored most ads in magazines. Some of the exotic items like the star fruit were expensive, but buying an eggplant wasn't going to bankrupt me. I had always stuck to the familiar fruits, the apples and bananas, because they were safe and comfortable and not purple. I couldn't recall eating anything purple. Wasn't that usually nature's warning sign *not* to eat something? I'd been eating healthy for about two years, and it was unlikely I was going to get completely derailed by a sudden obsession with mangos. It was time to widen my food horizons.

And I needed blogging material.

I decided I would "Lick the Produce." I wrote an entry every month about new foods I'd tried. I wasn't too upset that I'd lived a life without turnips, but after I ate some sweet-potato fries I realized life would have been sweeter with the tuberous roots in my life. I felt stupid when I realized eggplant was purple only on the outside, not the inside, and I'd actually eaten it many times in spaghetti sauce at the Olive Garden. I randomly picked items from the store even though I had no idea how to cook them. I relied on recipe websites to tell me what to chop off the green onions and how to scrape out a spaghetti squash. Grocers didn't print cooking instructions on the vegetables. This is why I steamed a dish full of radishes. The Internet made me do it.

My readers were quick to tell me that steaming radishes was a bit odd. I'd initially written them off as too bitter to try again. When I tried them as a garnish on a salad or roasted with soy sauce and olive oil, I was glad I'd given them a second chance. I wondered if the reason so many people hated eating vegetables was because they just didn't know how to prepare them correctly. I certainly hadn't.

I'd always assumed people who ate healthy food led miserable lives but didn't realize it, like all those people who used AOL. I thought people who shopped at organic grocery stores were granola-crunching hippies who never ate sugar or fat or anything that tasted good. When I was fat, I couldn't conceive that anyone could eat healthy foods all the time and enjoy it. I was wrong on two counts. First, this stuff tasted good even though it was good for me. Second, I still ate unhealthy food from time to time. I had once wished I was like a friend of mine who didn't like the taste of chocolate so I'd never have the urge to eat a bag of M&M's. But now I was glad I hadn't had our tongues swapped in a back alley surgery in Mexico. I ate foods that were part of a well-balanced diet, but I balanced that diet with small portions of sugar-rich, fat-filled sweets from time to time. Cutting treats out entirely wouldn't be very balanced. Everyone should be able to have a slice of her own birthday cake. Hell, she should have three.

I wasn't going to give up my enjoyment of food to become thin. I had once envied smokers and alcoholics because they got to eliminate their vices from their lives, whereas I would always have to eat. Now I realized I had the better end of the deal because I was managing to eat responsibly. I just hadn't done it all at once. I slowly introduced myself to all these new foods, just like I slowly switched my cat's food by blending it with his old kibble. If I had put him on his new prescription diet food all at once, I would have received an indignant glare and a poopy present at the foot of my bed. People were the same way. If I'd tried changing my diet all at once, I wouldn't have pooped on my bedspread, but I would have thrown a hissy fit.

As much as I now loved a dessert of fat-free vanilla yogurt topped with mango cornflake cereal, I had a distinct memory of hating vanilla yogurt as recently as high school. It had been too tart for my tastes. When I'd first switched to diet sodas I'd spent three weeks wondering if losing a couple of pounds was worth drinking liquid that tasted like drain water. Now I found regular sodas to be far too sweet. I'd heard the phrase "acquired taste" before, but now I was starting to realize what it meant. Just because something tasted different didn't mean it was bad. If I kept eating a food regularly, I often really started to like it after adjusting the flavor. (Brussel sprouts were not one of these items.) Once I stopped bombarding myself with sugar all the time, I started to appreciate subtler tastes that had been drowned out by all that corn syrup. I didn't even want sugar that much anymore. I glided past the bags of chocolate marshmallow pinwheels in the grocery store with only a half-second pause in my step.

I was collecting healthy recipes faster than I could actually cook them. I loved all the new taste experiences happening in my mouth. Just a little less than two years ago I'd resented every single minute I'd spent in front of the skillet grilling a chicken breast. Now I was spending up to half an hour or more preparing meals and had more than thirty pages of recipes in my binder. Cooking used to be a strange new activity; now it was just a normal part of my day. I was genuinely excited to learn how to roast cauliflower and grill zucchini. I dragged my mother to Bed, Bath and Beyond to show her the flexible wonder of silicone muffin pans.

Smack me with a spatula, I *liked* to cook.

The first inkling I was going mad was when I made a soufflé more than a year ago. I'd never made a food with its own accent mark. I don't know why my family hadn't had me committed when they saw me digging beneath the mismatched Tupperware containers without lids, searching for the mixer. Perhaps they were afraid I'd see the men in white coats holding out a straitjacket and attack them with beaters set to puree?

I had no idea what a soufflé was other than a food cooked on sitcoms solely for comedic value. It always collapsed after a character made a loud noise. Making a soufflé involved separating egg whites. That just *sounded* hard. I would never have made the attempt if my mother hadn't shown me the nifty gadget she had procured long ago, at a Tupperware party well before my birth, which easily separated the yolk from the whites.

When I beat the egg whites in the mixer they got frothy and stiff as the protein strands unraveled and formed structures around air molecules. They looked like frosting, which was a shame because they still tasted like eggs. I dutifully folded in some seasoned apples and let the concoction bake in the oven. It came out . . . okay. I'm sure my ambivalence had nothing to do with the burned edges around the top.

I was considering making the soufflé again just so I could use the egg white separator. I loved gadgets. A stroll through the kitchen section of the housewares store was like visiting a foreign culture. It was amazing how many devices I could buy that served only one purpose. They were like graduate students with overly specific dissertations. My absolute favorite gadget was the egg slicer. I loved to nestle a freshly boiled egg in the valley of its base and then pull the wire rack down through its tender body. The wires cut cleanly and easily through the white and the yolk, leaving perfectly circular slices. I could punch the yolk out like a hole puncher.

Cooking was also a good excuse to beat the crap out of things. After a bad day I didn't need to eat a bag of chocolate when I could smash out my feelings on a bag of clumpy frozen spinach. It was also cheaper than $200 an hour for a therapist. I was thinking of getting a meat hammer so I could whale on some fat chicken breasts in the name of faster cooking times. And I loved my big knife; it was as long as my forearm and looked like it had been stolen from the set of a slasher movie. I felt so powerful, effortlessly slicing through zucchini skin. Plus, I didn't need to fear prowlers.

Recipes also appealed to the computer geek in me because they were open source. When I bought a recipe book, I got the source code for the food—as the chef, I could compile the recipe as written into the final product, but since I also had the code, I could make changes to suit myself, add subroutines or variables by sprinkling in extra ingredients. As in the software world, some food was closed source, such as the recipe for Pepsi or KFC's blend of herbs and spices. However, you could always try reverse engineering the recipe yourself.

As I experimented in the kitchen, I learned how to slightly alter recipes. It was similar to how I learned programming techniques during my day job as a web developer. After sampling some tasty mint-chocolate fudge pudding at a friend's house, I was tempted to buy more, but I scoffed at the price of pudding cups. It was cheaper to buy the dry mix, but it didn't come in the chocolate-mint flavor. I figured all I needed was some mint extract, which I dumped into a regular batch of chocolate pudding. I licked a wobbly lump off the spoon and it tasted amazing. I was shocked. I was more shocked when I licked the teaspoon after measuring the mint extract and experienced the taste equivalent of looking directly at the sun. On the bright side, I would never have to buy mouthwash again.

Real foodies probably consider this stuff second nature, but it had never occurred to me that you could make up your own recipes. I imagined recipes had been perfectly chiseled on stone tablets and handed down to us by God. How had anyone figured out how to make something as complicated as bread? Even my failed food experiments were somewhat rewarding because they allowed me to be creative in a task I had otherwise found routine and tedious. I used to secretly snicker at women who proudly displayed their prize-winning bundt cakes on morning talk shows, but now I realized that cooking was an outlet to express creativity just like painting or music. Flour, shortening, and sugar were more likely to be found in a housewife's home than oil paints and canvas.

Ironically, I knew more about cooking now than I ever had when I was fat. I needed to keep trying new foods to keep myself interested. I didn't want to get in a rut and go back to my old ways out of boredom. I was applying this same strategy outside of the kitchen too.

I weighed about 210 pounds now, which on a five-foot-nine woman was only eight pounds away from being considered overweight instead of obese. When I'd first started exercising the only thing my joints could handle was walking. If I'd tried breaking into a run I would have found myself wailing by the back of the treadmill, grasping my knee in pain like Nancy Kerrigan and shouting, "Why me?!" But now my body could actually do things.

I'd started testing the limits of my abilities one year into my weight loss, in January of 2006 when I weighed 245 pounds. I tried following an aerobics video that was so old I owned it on VHS instead of DVD. An energetic female instructor told me I'd have lots of fun bouncing along to some Motown favorites. I had first tried to groove with her when I'd weighed 350-something pounds. Back then I would hit the stop button only seven minutes into the tape, and that included the thirty seconds of FBI warning. I had realized there was no way I could move as fast as the exercisers on the video, and I tossed the tape back on the shelf.

When I inserted the tape this time, I watched the tracking automatically adjust the horizontal line of static off the screen and guessed I wouldn't last much longer than seven minutes. Twenty-six minutes later I hit the stop button, and not because I'd collapsed on the remote control. I wasn't even physically exhausted yet, just too frustrated to learn the steps. I still hadn't watched that tape all the way through. There could have been porn at the end, and I'd have been none the wiser.

This was amazing. I'd seen progress in the decreasing sizes on my clothes tags, but now I had proof that I was actually getting more fit. I'd spent a year walking nowhere on the treadmill, but I was definitely getting somewhere.

But aerobics still didn't appeal to me. I needed something to add to my routine other than walking or I might quit out of boredom. I tried Pilates the next month. It was supposed to improve my posture and flexibility and give me a cute butt. Some other weight-loss bloggers had been talking about it, so I thought I'd give it a try. I spent $20 on a DVD, bought a mat, and started miming visits to the gynecologist's office on the living-room floor every other day for months. I looked absolutely ridiculous, rolling around on my huge ass. The instructor told me to scoop out my abdominals like I was leaning over a beach ball, which wasn't hard to imagine since my front pouch resembled one. Pilates helped me shed any scrap of dignity I was clinging to. Once I accepted that I was going to look like an utter fool whenever I tried something new, I felt free to do basically whatever I wanted. Pilates also kicked my ass, or more accurately my abs. Two days after bending my body in positions I had never before attempted or known possible, it hurt to laugh, sneeze, or moan in pain.

I loved it.

If I were this sore, something had to be working. Some Pilates moves were cute, such as "The Seal," which required me to clap my legs together three times and roll backward to clap them again. I threw in a couple of "arf, arfs" for fun. At first I had to do modified versions of the moves, bending my legs instead of fully extending them. I would roll only halfway backward instead of all the way to my shoulders. I had started stumbling through the routine at the end of February, but by the beginning of September I could do everything, including the teaser, or as I liked to call it, the motherfucking teaser. If there were ever a pose of the human body that required profanity, it was this one. I started lying down with my legs aimed toward the ceiling at a forty-five degree angle and my arms stretched out above my head. Then I sat up like the letter V for victory, my ass as the fulcrum, arms extended forward. I held the pose and then lay back down. I repeated the moves six times and collapsed.

I had never felt so awesome in my life. Surely it wouldn't be too long before I was bending like a pretzel and cramming myself into a pickle jar for my audition for the Cirque du Soleil.

Later, when I had started to enjoy my time in the kitchen mutilating yellow squash, I decided it was time I finally started lifting weights. I'd talked about lifting weights forever. I'd even followed a half-assed routine a year ago without doing much research. I'd quit after a month. I had been eating fewer calories than I was burning, but since I hadn't been strength training, part of the weight I'd lost was muscle, not fat. My body metabolized what it decided I could spare, and if I wasn't using my muscles, they were fair game. This was bad. I didn't want to lose muscle mass because it burned calories even when it was just sitting around, like my cell phone drained my battery just by being turned on. If I built more muscle, my metabolism would speed up and I could eat more. That sounded great to me.

I would build muscle by lifting heavy dumbbells, which would make tiny tears in my muscle tissue. I would rest a day or two to give my muscle time to repair itself and grow bigger and stronger. I ate some protein and carbs right after my workout to give my body the materials to complete these repairs. It was a great excuse to eat three sweet-potato muffins. I would then repeat the process, slowly increasing my weights and the number of repetitions. Destroy, then rebuild. Destroy and rebuild again, like Rome.

But lifting heavy things was hard. And it hurt. And it made my weight plateau. Muscle is more dense than fat. Muscle is like a box of books and fat is a box of pillows. Which one would you rather carry up the stairs? Muscle is more compact than fat, so even though my weight was staying the same, I was getting leaner and more shapely. The scale was just too dumb to realize that. Thankfully I'd witnessed the scale weave back and forth like a drunken driver before. I didn't enjoy the stall-out, but I wasn't crushed by it.

I wanted a more toned, fit body, but I didn't want to be as buff as Linda Hamilton in *Terminator 2*. I wouldn't have to fight killer cyborgs from the future . . . as far as I knew. I wasn't going to get huge muscles because women simply don't have enough testosterone to become as ripped as men without drugs or supplements. As long as I avoided gamma bomb blasts and kept a cool temper, I wouldn't end up looking like the She-Hulk.

After three months of training I flexed my arms in the mirror and was astonished by the pleasing curves I saw. My shoulders were so round, my collarbones so defined, my armpits so hard to shave. Damn those pectoral muscles! I would have wondered if I'd had an arm transplant if not for the hanging underarm flab. I was going to enjoy showing off my new arms in the sleeveless dress I'd bought for my older brother's wedding.

Who needed sleeves when you had awesome biceps?

I made a vow to keep trying new activities. I signed up for a kickboxing aerobics class offered through my county's school system. I flailed through the kickboxing routines five seconds behind everybody else. I almost knocked out my classmate with a poorly controlled roundhouse kick, and she hadn't even done anything to piss me off. I totally sucked, but I kept going to classes and eventually learned the difference between a hook and an upper cut. I'd never taken an aerobics class before, but I loved kicking and punching to cheesy techno songs. My small boobs were actually an asset because I wasn't knocked unconscious by bouncing globes when I did jumping jacks.

I was able to do all the crunches even though other people were flopping on their mats like trout on a boat deck. At the end of class we stretched on our mats. I'd been doing Pilates long enough that I could lie on my back and point my left leg toward the ceiling while the right leg lay flat on the mat at a ninety-degree angle. I noticed most of the other students had to bend their right legs to achieve the position. I smiled secretly in smug superiority. Then I turned my head to the left. The woman next to me had her right leg flat on the mat and her left leg bent straight back *behind her head*. Clearly, her muscles and ligaments had been replaced by rubber bands. Suddenly I didn't feel so superior.

Once that class ended, I signed up for tennis lessons. I was idly considering buying some in-line skates too after observing the skaters on the trail. It might be fun, assuming I didn't lose control, slam into the red bridge rail, and tumble ass over end into the river. After that, maybe I'd try martial arts? I'd probably watched way too much *Buffy* and *Xena* and *La Femme Nikita* on TV, but ass kicking looked like fun. By the time I was sixty maybe I'd get around to the luge.

I had been tricked. I'd started all this healthy eating and exercising only so I could get what I wanted—thin. Now I was actually enjoying it. It was like the time I'd tried a free trial of Netflix thinking I could get a free month's worth of DVDs and then quit once I'd gotten my free rentals. Now I had hundreds of movies in my queue and would never be able to watch them as quickly as I added them. Thank goodness I'd never joined a bug-eating club. I might find myself swatting flies, dipping them in Dijon mustard sauce, and enjoying it.

Weight loss in itself was a somewhat empty reward. All the cool things that I could do because of my new fitness and health were the real prize. The buzz of fitting into a new dress size and seeing the descending numbers on the scale was a great high, but eventually it wore off. Now I could get a runner's high several times a week. A year after I'd first run a mile I was still ecstatic that I could run that far without being chased by a bear. I was thinking less like a dieter and more like an athlete. I certainly was starting to feel like one. I owned *two* sports bras now. I wanted to try everything. I wanted to see what this new body could do.

For most of my life I had considered my body the transportation vehicle for my brain—a head attached to a torso with arms and legs was fine, but if I had to stick my brain in a jar and scuttle around on robotic spider legs I would have managed. My internal world was the important one, not the external.

In college our teaching assistant had walked into the psychology lab one day carrying a human brain in a jar. He wasn't a psycho killer. The brain had been donated to science, which evidently meant to us. Everyone in the small classroom pushed aside cheap plastic chairs to gather around the brain sitting on a folding table. The dull gray organ floated like a bath toy in the preservative fluid. It looked just like a movie prop. I lasted about ten seconds before I was hit with a wave of nausea and pulled back to my chair in the undertow.

Typically I was squeamish around blood and human organs, but that wasn't the cause of my sickness. That brain had belonged to a real human being; it had stored all his memories, processed all his thoughts, enabled his entire being. And now a bunch of freshmen were gawking over it on their way to four credit hours. Everything that made him himself was now encapsulated in a piece of organic matter that could be easily squished if an underclassman got clumsy with the jar. I might have considered my mind to be the most important part of me, but as I stared at the brain, I faced the reality that it was just as fleshy and vulnerable as my skin, as breakable as my bones.

As I became more and more fit, I started to realize that my brain and my body were not separate entities that could be ripped apart. My brain required nutrients and chemicals to run properly, just as a car required gas and oil to run. When I was eating well and exercising, my mind functioned better. I could focus for longer periods and think more clearly. Ultimately I was just a collection of molecules powered by small electrical currents. If I fed myself the proper nutrients and stimulated the release of healthy chemicals via exercise, my body and my mind ran better.

I wondered why I had to come to this realization on my own when it should have been covered in health class or PE. I had thought physical education was pointless. I went to school to be educated, not to feel inferior because I couldn't climb the rope. When would I ever need to climb a rope, anyway? When I read an article about a middle school teacher in Pensacola, Florida, who let kids out of gym class for a dollar a day, I was immediately envious that my PE teachers hadn't been so entrepreneurial.[1]

Of course, maybe they had been and I never heard about it because I was so good at avoiding gym class. In middle school, I learned how to play flute so I could take band during gym period. In high school, I was required to take only one semester of gym, which I took during summer school so I could cram more electives into my regular schedule. I attended every day, four hours a day, for four weeks. The suffering was condensed into bite-size portions that took up one-sixth of my day. But there was also a fear that had nothing to do with my inability to serve a volleyball over the net. If I missed more than two classes, I'd have to take the whole course over again because of absenteeism. The only thing more horrible than gym class was the thought of taking gym class twice.

It's a shame that none of my physical education teachers were able to convince me that being fit could be fun or that it could enhance other aspects of my life. Instead, gym was about the fear of group showering and avoiding dodge balls. Gym was about being picked on for being weak. Now that I wasn't being screamed at by a blond with a mullet wearing track pants, I could see that my physical health directly affected my mood and my ability to think. A healthy lifestyle made my body feel better. It made my body *look* much better too.

It also made my body more useful. I could now run quickly to the corner to cross the street before the walk signal flashed red. I could carry twenty-four-packs of soda up the driveway and into the house without panting. I felt powerful, and I hadn't had to usurp any South American nations or run for political office to feel this power. Fitness gave me confidence that bled into all areas of my life, not just those involving volleyball nets.

I felt confident enough to sign up for a 5K race. The former-fat-girl bylaws dictate that you must run a 5K or you will be forced to gain back all the weight. On the day of the run I was handed my T-shirt and a map of the race course. The map's red line ran by the lawn at White River State Park and the zoo parking lot that I had barely been able to walk to after a concert three years ago. As I ran through the streets, passing fluorescent pylons and dodging paper water cups tossed to the ground, I imagined overlaying this moment with the past to overlap time in a split screen. I broke my stride for a second to wave at that fat girl who struggled to walk half as fast as I was running now, but she didn't see me. She kept her head down and staggered forward with labored breaths, hoping she could make it another hundred yards and down the concrete steps. I breathed heavily too, miles more to go. I stepped up my pace and passed her by.

CHAPTER 15

Decloaking

"**W**ow, you look really great!" my dental hygienist said as I stared into the light hovering above me like an alien spaceship. Visiting the dentist *was* like being probed by aliens.

"Yeah, I've lost a lot of weight," I replied, resting my clasped hands gently on my stomach. Two years ago I had grasped my hands tightly together as gravity pulled my heavy arms in opposite directions down the steep slope of my belly. Today they lay relaxed on my slightly rounded stomach even when I released my grip.

"I noticed," the hygienist said.

My dental care provider had been very tactful. She hadn't directly addressed my weight but had left the door open if I wanted to enter the room of that particular conversation. Smooth. They must have taught that technique during "Small Talk 101" in dental school, where they also covered how to make conversation with people with a dozen cotton swabs stuck in their gums.

"How much weight have you lost?" she asked as she reached for a shiny tool on her tray.

"Um . . ." I rolled my eyes upward as if the response were written on the bottom of my eyelashes. The answer to this question kept changing, and I couldn't remember what the proper number was this month. My starting weight of 372 minus my current weight of 197 would make it . . .

"One hundred and seventy-five," I replied, proud that I could do the mental math. "I weigh about 195 pounds now." I sounded like such a liar. That number was absurd. How could I have been able to walk around with that much extra weight? I could barely carry my TV set up the stairs. The last two years must have been a fever dream occurring in a diabetic coma after I'd finally eaten too much frosting straight from the jar. When I'd lost only twenty to thirty pounds, I'd told everyone from the janitor to the deli waiter. Now I'd lost so much that it was becoming uncomfortable to mention. It was freakish. It sounded like I was bragging. I'd received so many compliments about my weight loss by friends, family, and blog readers that I'd reached a saturation point. I didn't feel a need to fish for positive reinforcement anymore.

"Wow," she said, her eyes wider and rounder than the mirror tool she held in her hand. "That's amazing! That's more than I weigh! You should be proud," she said as she continued to pick plaque off my gum line.

"Thanks," I mumbled without moving my jaw. It had been about two years since I'd popped a can of soda pop that didn't have the word "diet" on it. My body mass index now qualified me as overweight instead of obese. It made sense that the dental staff would be particularly impressed by my transformation. They saw me only every six months, so it was as if they were viewing time-lapse photography. They saw me in a strobe light that flickered every six months.

I was getting better at these exchanges about my weight. They weren't that different from all the other scripts I practiced in life. When someone said, "How are you doing today?" in the hallway I'd reply, "Just fine!" even if I wanted to crawl back into my bed and drool on the pillows. If someone congratulated me on my weight loss, I'd just say thanks and smile. People were rather predictable. There were only so many ways they reacted to my metamorphosis.

I preferred it when people simply said I looked good without specifically mentioning my weight. I could look great for many reasons—because I got a haircut, because I was wearing a cute blouse, or because it was a sunny day and I felt happy. Someone who said, "You look great since you lost all that weight" was implying I had not looked so great before. It was as close as you could come to building a time machine and traveling to the past to insult me.

The hygienist finished scraping my teeth and set the tool down in favor of the electric polisher and a tray of polishing paste. "You know, I would never have guessed you weighed 195. You look a lot thinner than that. Mint, strawberry, or piña colada?"

"Yeah, it was a lot. Piña colada." I replied.

People were terrible at guessing my weight. Before I got too fat to ride the roller coasters, I bought a season pass to an amusement park for the summer and noticed a "Guess My Weight" game positioned in the thoroughfare. It was right next to the walkway over the highway, which granted it maximum crowd exposure and unlimited opportunity for embarrassment. Next to the barker was a scale with a circular face so large it could have doubled as Godzilla's Frisbee. The barker had to guess your weight within five or ten pounds or you'd win a prize.

I never played this game. Public weigh-ins seemed reserved for the sanctity of Weight Watchers meetings, which I'd never attended since I was a diet atheist. I didn't know how much I weighed, and I didn't want to find out in front of packs of teenyboppers in short-shorts sucking down Diet Coke and Dippin' Dots. However, I *was* curious to know how well the barker could guess someone's weight. Most people didn't stand next to a humongous scale all day. If I were brave enough to risk insulting someone by guessing his or her weight, I couldn't be sure that I was getting accurate feedback. Surely most people lied anyway. Without a huge scale you couldn't know how wrong you were and make corrections in the future.

Recently Kirstie Alley had been on *Oprah* in a bikini, and one blogger said she must be lying about her weight. The blogger was about the same size as Kirstie and weighed more. I had no idea what Kirstie Alley really weighed. I did know that when you factored in height differences, ratio of fat to muscle, and other nonsense like how much sodium you'd had recently and when your last trip to the bathroom was, you couldn't assume someone on TV weighed as much as you did just because she looked the same size.

People always seemed scared of guessing that I weighed more than 200 pounds. Nobody would even touch 300. Instead they copped for numbers right below the threshold. It was as if 200 were the magical fat number. At 199 you were still thin, but if you rolled over to 200 you had passed the point of no return. No one dared guess a number near my actual highest weight, perhaps because they feared insulting me. I wondered if the carnival barker made adjustments to avoid being mauled by angry fat people. If he thought someone actually weighed 205, would he round down to 199? How could I know if the carnival scale was even calibrated accurately? Carnies were notoriously stingy about giving away their pink teddy bears.

I had read that people became increasingly worse at estimating amounts the larger portions became.[1] Most people can guess the calorie content of a small meal with little error, but if you stacked more and more ribs and potatoes on a plate you underestimated the calorie content by more and more too. Perhaps the same was true with weight.

The hygienist sprayed some water in my mouth. I swished the remains of my piña colada paste until she stuck the suction tube in my mouth. "The doctor will be by in a couple of minutes to check for cavities," she said, writing some notes on my chart.

"Okay," I said as she elevated the chair to a sitting position.

"So what have you been doing?" she asked. "To lose weight, I mean."

I didn't want to say I was on a diet because I hated that word. It sounded as if I were eating only rice cakes and tofu until the day I could finally fit into a size 4 dress, at which time I'd resume eating chocolate fudge brownies for breakfast. It belied the significance of the commitment that I'd made to living a new lifestyle, as if I were calling my two-year marriage with healthy living a "fling." But there was no other word to use. It was such a mouthful to say I was living a new lifestyle and it sounded pretentious too. I was *sort of* on a diet because I was following some general guidelines, but they weren't restricting my enjoyment of life or food in any significant way.

"Oh, I've been cutting out white flour, sugars, stuff like that. Eating more vegetables." How could I possibly sum up everything I'd been doing in a succinct small-talk paragraph? I hated trying to simplify everything, but I doubted she wanted to hear my hour-long lecture on Weight Loss 101. Instead I came off sounding like an idiot who told people to eat less and move more. If only it had been that simple.

She nodded. "My aunt has been doing that too. She says it's remarkable how much better she feels."

"Oh yeah, it's kind of amazing. It's a world of difference. I really love it," I said. Oh no. I had become one of those women who talked about her diet. Frequently women had tried to bond with me by talking about what they were eating or how much they hated their bodies. It was called fat talk. I wanted it banned.

At a funeral luncheon I'd attended, a woman across the table started lobbing potato salad and chips onto her paper plate as I picked fruit off a serving tray. We made eye contact. "I keep saying I'm going to go on a diet, but I keep putting it off," she said out of nowhere. I quickly glanced up and down her body and determined she wasn't fat. "Yep," she continued. "Got to go on a diet. Any day now."

I hoped that if I ever started talking like this woman, someone would drown me in the punch bowl. I didn't care what she was eating. I didn't care what she looked like. I didn't care if she greased her tummy with butter wedges and belly-slid down the table to catch slices of German chocolate cake and raspberry cheesecake in her mouth. It surely would have livened up the affair.

I didn't know why she felt the need to apologize for eating and enjoying food. It seemed as if she were saying she was sorry she wasn't thin enough or good enough. It sounded like she was insulting herself. Why did so many women relate to each other this way? Being dissatisfied with your body was more of a requirement to be female than possessing a vagina. Occasionally thin friends had whined to me about how fat they were when I was still at a size that I struggled to buckle myself into the front seat of the car. They were fat? Had they not noticed I needed a seat belt extender? I think they were so used to obsessing about their fat with friends that they automatically did the same thing with me.

The odd thing about fat talk was that it became less acceptable the fatter I became. If a thin friend talked about how fat she was, it wasn't a matter of life and death, but for me it was. If I said I needed to go on a diet it wasn't just a flippant, self-hating remark but a serious and uncomfortable topic of conversation. I doubted this church lady would have yammered on about needing to go on a diet if my thighs were still as big as her torso. Fat was only okay to talk about if you didn't have any on your body.

I didn't like talking about diets with other women, like my dental hygienist, because there was the strong implication that we should all be on one, as though we could never be thin enough or good enough or possibly be happy with how we looked, so we'd better watch what went in our mouths. God forbid that we actually enjoy what we were eating. If you dared to eat a donut you'd better be prepared to do penance at the gym. That wasn't how I felt at all. I was still technically fat, but I thought I looked rather awesome. I ate foods that I enjoyed and paid attention to what I was eating, but I had started eating healthy so I could live longer. I didn't want eating healthy to become my life.

"I wish I could just lose these last fifteen pounds," the hygienist said as my eyes searched for the dentist. There were no telltale screams or drilling noises to give away his location. "You make me feel like such a slacker."

I now inspired more shame in people than priests. I listened to all their food confessions. Too bad I couldn't tell them to say ten Hail Marys to wash away their dieting sins. I could try empathizing with her and say the first hundred pounds were a lot easier than the second hundred, but that sounded flippant. I thought about patting her shoulder and saying, "That's too bad." I was never sure if these self-derogatory comments were a backhanded way of seeking tips. I didn't have any advice on how to lose the last fifteen pounds because I hadn't lost the last fifteen pounds yet. I was starting to become thinner than some of my friends, however. One of them dug her elliptical machine out of the basement in fear when she saw I was going to pass her on the way down the scales. I'd felt the same way when I had been fat and read an article about all the weight the thousand-pound man had lost and realized he was going to catch up with me.

I felt my own hints of guilt when I encountered overweight friends. I didn't want to make them feel bad about themselves, but I wasn't going to gain weight again just to make them feel better. I was careful to try not to brag about how much I'd lost or to mention food or exercise around them. When my best friend had complimented me on my weight loss and told me she was proud of me, I'd tried to downplay it and said, "Well, I'm still technically fat." I thought it was preferable to saying, "I am the most awesome person on the planet. Bow down before me and balance this bowl of seedless grapes on your head."

I was actually glad to see the dentist as he plopped down on the rotating stool next to my chair, ending my conversation about the evils of white flour. I passed the checkup without the discovery of any new cavities and made my way out to the lobby to pay my bill. As I waited in line behind another patient, the wooden door swung open and another hygienist popped her head out.

"Hey, I wanted to tell you how great you look!" she said.

"Thanks," I said. Smile. Head tilt. I was getting *so* good at this.

"What have you been doing?" she inquired. The man in line flashed me a curious glance.

"I changed my diet and I've been doing a lot of walking," I said, again trying to simplify my life into a twelve-word sentence.

"That's it?" She gave me a surprised look.

"Basically, yeah." The man in front of me finished paying and left. I approached the counter.

"Wow! That's fantastic!" she said, taken aback. "Congratulations!"

"Thanks," I said. Smile. I could take this show on the road.

She closed the door and left. As I waited for the credit-card machine to print out the slip for me to sign, I wondered if the hygienist had expected me to say "weight-loss surgery" when answering her question. The increasing popularity of weight-loss surgery was making it unusual for someone to lose almost two hundred pounds the old-fashioned way. It was a shame that strangers assumed it was the only answer. I didn't particularly mind if they thought I'd had surgery, but it seemed to impress people a lot more when they found out I hadn't. I was glad I'd avoided going under the knife, but I didn't think I deserved extra credit for it, although everyone else did.

I don't know how I would view what I had done if it had happened to someone else. I hoped I'd just be happy for her and not judge how she'd gone about it. If the whole dieting and exercise thing hadn't worked out, I probably would have been counting backward from one hundred on a surgeon's table in another ten years. If something had gone awry during my early transitioning stages, I could easily have been testing the weight limits of the dentist's chair during my appointment. I wasn't a better person simply because I'd figured out how to lose a lot of weight without a surgeon's intervention. I wasn't sure I completely understood how I'd done it, anyway.

I *was* proud of all my hard work. Weight loss was something I had made happen, not something that had happened to me. I wasn't sure that I'd feel the same way if I'd had surgery. I felt really comfortable in my body despite the drastic remodeling it had undergone. Two years ago I had suspected that I would always feel like a fat girl even when I lost all the weight. Strangely, I didn't feel that way at all. I felt in control of my transformation. It wasn't like someone had mugged me on the street and stolen all my fat.

But I had mixed feelings about all the compliments I was getting. People looked at me and saw only what wasn't there. I had worked very hard, worked my ass off, in fact, but people were acting like I'd just juggled flaming bananas with my toes while blindfolded. Weight loss was hard work, but was being fat such a bad thing to be?

Back when I was fat, a coworker had brought in pictures of her new granddaughter to show everyone at the call center. Everyone crowded around the photos, glad to have an excuse to stop asking people on the other end of the line about their detergent preferences. "She's beautiful!" they said. "Such a pretty one!" another woman cooed. "Gorgeous eyes, and a cute nose too." This kid couldn't even control her bowel movements, but her life was already made. She was pretty and people loved her for it. Granted, she was a bit young to be complimented for her jump shot or her math skills, but I had noticed that people on game shows never talked about their fat and ugly kids during their twenty-second interviews. Pretty was power. I wondered if the strangers I had called on the phone about their buying habits heard my alto voice and thought I was a slender and sexy girl instead of a woman with her ass spilling out of her seat. I might not have been stripper material, but I probably could have gotten phone sex work.

As a child I had denied that looks were important. In my adolescence I became angry at everyone who discriminated against me because of my appearance. Now I'd just accepted that pretty, thin people were treated better. It was easiest if I just tried to manipulate that to my best advantage. I felt funny at first, admitting that one reason I wanted to lose weight was because I *did* care about my looks and I *did* care about what people thought. I wanted to be above all that shallow nonsense. But I wasn't immune to looks discrimination myself. When I saw a man with creepy eyes and arched eyebrows in the hallway, I had to remind myself that bushy brows didn't necessarily mean he was a serial killer. I suspected part of the human brain was permanently wired to make judgments about people based on their looks. I could only acknowledge my biases and do my best to work around them. Fat people weren't the only ones who got treated differently because of how they looked. My five-foot-one friend got patted on the head by strangers who thought her height was cute, although her personality had more bite than her petite frame implied.

If I were to tape-record all these compliments and play them backward on a tape maybe I'd hear a secret message that said, "Thank you for conforming!" I was becoming thin now. I was blending in. I was living up to the expectation that I become a slender, socially acceptable female. I was starting to reap the benefits of thin privilege. When a thin, young, white girl had gone missing in Aruba last year, I had gotten sick of watching the news coverage because I knew that Nancy Grace wouldn't have sent a search party after my fat ass. Now I was thin enough that my disappearance might warrant a spot on a news crawl at the bottom of the screen. This wasn't something I was proud of, but it was making my life easier. I *could* be proud that it wasn't the driving reason behind my new lifestyle. I felt so good lately. The weight loss was starting to seem incidental. If I never lost another pound but still got to feel this fit and powerful, I could deal with it.

As I walked through the lobby to exit the building, an obese woman in a baggy blouse and black pants entered through the door with a jingle of the bell. She was out of breath from the walk across the parking lot and looked tired. I was suddenly flooded with relief. *Thank God I'm not like that anymore,* I thought. The limited mobility. The public shame. The restricted clothing options. Been there. Done that. Still had the fat pants. I never wanted those pants to fit again.

I passed by her and smiled as I left. She didn't know I used to be bigger than her. I felt like I was in the obesity witness protection program. I had always been fat, but now I wasn't. It was a gigantic issue that had shaped who I was, physically and as a person. Now people didn't have to know unless I told them. Skinny actors who played fat people in movies got to take their fat suits off at the end of the day and go back to their lives. I was taking mine off and returning to a life I hadn't quite had before.

I wanted to tell her about how I had changed, that I had become more than I was, and less, all at the same time. But I just averted my eyes and headed for the parking lot. I didn't want to be like the family I had walked past on the trail who handed me a flyer asking if I had accepted Jesus Christ as my personal savior. I didn't need to save all the fat girls of the world. My own relationship with my body had nothing to do with hers. I wasn't Mother Teresa to the chubby.

Not everyone felt that same way about me, though. I got an anonymous comment on the blog that said I would never be the "equal" of naturally thin people because I could never be "permanently or safety [sic] thin." Anonymous sounded really bitter. Usually people who felt secure about their bodies didn't feel the need to leave snide comments on weight-loss blogs. I guessed Anonymous was either a thin person who thought his size was the only thing going for him or a fat person who wanted to be thin but couldn't. Now he went around telling fat people it was impossible to lose weight so he could feel better about himself. He would probably throw a pizza party if I ever regained the weight because it would prove his own fatalistic philosophy correct. It really aggravated some people if you did something they thought was impossible.

I decided to keep the weight off just to piss him off. Health and mobility were good reasons too, but weight loss as vengeance had more fire and brimstone. The best revenge would be to live happily ever after.

Some scientists believed that the reduced obese, as I was now called, were metabolically different from people who had never been fat.[2] Some studies suggested I would burn 15 percent fewer calories when I exercised because my body was trying to get back to my fatter set point. I didn't know if this were true or not, but if I had to run 15 percent farther every day, so be it. It sucked. It wasn't fair. Oh well, I never got that pony I wanted as a little girl either. I *had* gotten more fat cells than people who'd always been thin. Once my fat cells reached a certain threshold size, they stimulated the creation of new fat cells that would never go away.[3] In this sense, I *was* different.

But the anonymous coward's comments seemed to imply that thin people were lumped into two groups: The formerly fat were the nouveau riche, but the always slender had old money they'd invested in thin stocks decades ago. This seemed ridiculous to me. Sure, I was still learning how to navigate people's changed perceptions of me as a skinny person, but that didn't mean I was only passing for thin. Honestly, I was still fat-ish.

But I thought of myself as a thin person, which was all that seemed to matter. To some extent, being fat was a state of mind. Fat was a way you could feel as well as a description of yourself. I thought of Felicity, my high school friend who was thinner than I had ever been, and how she berated herself for her imaginary chub. I knew I still weighed more than she had, but I felt thinner than she ever had. I didn't feel as if I needed to act a certain way because of my size anymore. There was no need to hide in my room or cover up my arm flab. I was much more acceptable to the world in my current form, but I cared less about what they thought than ever before. My new attitude was like a comb I'd gotten after all my hair had fallen out.

A couple of days later I needed to upgrade my cell phone plan. My phone was one of the models the cavemen had used to call their wives and ask if they felt like a woolly mammoth or saber-toothed tiger for dinner. My provider was going to cut off my service at the end of the year if I didn't get a new phone. I entered the mall through the second-floor walkway from the parking garage. I turned the corner quickly to escape the siren smell of the Cinnabon store only to be faced with a woman clothed in tackiness. Leopard-print leggings clung tightly to her legs and she strode confidently forward on suede boots with three-inch heels. She wore a red leather jacket over a black tank top, all topped off with frizzy blond hair in a ponytail held back with a leopard-print scrunchy. She looked equal parts awful and ridiculous.

As I strode forward, I took a step back mentally. I didn't have any right to judge what this woman was wearing. I might think she looked as if she had skinned a polyester cheetah, but I could tell from the swagger in her step that she felt good about herself. A fat girl who dared venture into the food court in a tank top would risk similar judgments from onlookers, but she would have every right to bare arms. No one had a right to say, "You shouldn't wear that," as long as your outfit didn't violate public decency laws. I admired the tacky woman's boldness, even if I didn't admire her outerwear.

I entered the cell phone store and approached the counter where a thin salesgirl in a frumpy polo shirt and ponytail stood. "Hello, can I help you?" she said in a soft voice. I handed her my coupon for a free phone and explained my problem. She began working to change my service plan, focusing mostly on the computer and avoiding eye contact. She reached a point on her computer screen where she didn't know what to do and needed help.

"Just a minute," she said. She turned and walked halfway across the store to where her manager was talking to another customer. She hovered behind him, afraid to interrupt, though they were not that deep in conversation. I picked up a pamphlet on the counter and started to read about their extensive coverage area. I read every single word of copy in the brochure. I was mildly disappointed the writers hadn't hidden any secret messages in it on the assumption no one would ever read it. I sighed and looked back across the store.

The girl was still hovering, head down and shoulders hunched. "Speak up!" I wanted to yell. She was passive and afraid to be seen. I used to be just like that. It was such fat-girl behavior, as if she were embarrassed to be taking up space. It was incredibly annoying. I had never liked being in those situations when I was the shy person, but it never occurred to me how sad it was to watch someone act like a wimp.

Eventually the manager finished the transaction with the other customer and helped the salesgirl finish my upgrade. I walked out of the store thinking about all the time I had wasted waiting to be noticed. But I was decloaking now, like a Romulan Bird of Prey on *Star Trek*, materializing off the port side and ready to fire my phasers. When I'd been fat, the gravity well formed by my mass might have caused light to bend around me, making me invisible. Not anymore.

I may have been smaller than I'd ever been, but I was ready to take up space in the world.

CHAPTER 16

Half-Assed

The liquor store clerk looked at my ID, then at my face, then at my ID again. After a slight hesitation he rung up my raspberry vodka, and I sighed in relief. It would still be another few months before I could renew my driver's license, but until then I'd have to deal with triple takes from alcohol salesmen and bouncers after they inspected the photo of me at my fattest, taken under fluorescent lights. Sometimes I'd pretended to have a skinnier sister. Now I seemed to be her.

Half of me was gone. I had finally done it. One hundred and eighty-six pounds were lost, hopefully never to be found again, which according to my driver's license meant I now weighed sixty-four pounds. After a little more than two years, one day I woke up, went to the bathroom, stepped on the scale, and the magic three numbers rolled up like three cherries on a slot machine. Jackpot!

I commemorated the event by taking a photo of myself standing in one leg of my fat pants. I used my camera timer, so I had to use my new athletic abilities to hop across my kitchen, pivot, and smile in less than ten seconds without slipping on the linoleum and cracking my skull on the stainless steel sink. At least I was prepared for the Potato

Sack Racing World Championships, should they ever be held. I invited all my blog readers to that party in my fat pants. There certainly was room for everyone.

So was I officially thin now? No one had waved a checkered flag as I'd hopped across my kitchen. My body mass index was 27.5, which was solidly "overweight," equidistant from being categorized as either "normal" or "obese." Would I be thin when I could no longer shop at the plus-size stores? Would it be when my body fat percentage was 25 percent? Surely I would be thin by the time my boobs finally stuck out farther than my belly, though at the rate the twins were decreasing that might never happen. When I stuck a pencil under my front flap of fat, it clattered to the floor instead of clinging above my pubic hair. By Hollywood standards I was still a fat ass, but I was on the thin side for a Botticelli beauty.

Most of the things that sucked about being a fat person had disappeared from my life. When I visited my older brother in Boston, I traipsed up and down the Freedom Trail, through a park by the harbor, and back to the train without panting like a Labrador. The next day I toured Cambridge with a skinnier friend from high school and secretly smiled when he said he was tired of walking, though I knew I could go for another mile or two.

The hallway to the elevators in my brother's apartment complex was coated in mirrors. Mirrors on the left, mirrors at the end; there was even a mirror on the ceiling of the elevator. I guessed this was some sort of vampire detection system. I checked out my image whenever we were coming or going. Each time I thought, *Damn, I look good.* It was great not being disgusted by my image. I highly recommend it. When we flew back home I didn't have to ask for a seat belt extender. I didn't feel like a fat person anymore. My life was no longer like a fat person's, but there was some residue. There was the skin.

Everyone wanted to know about the state of my skin. I felt like the spokeswoman for Neutrogena. It was a taboo subject to bring up, so my blog readers typically asked about it via email instead of leaving a comment publicly on the blog. They would usually tack on the qualifier that I didn't have to talk about it if it were too personal. I didn't consider it that personal of a question, any more so than if I were to ask, "How are your kidneys today? Still filtering waste products? Good to hear!"

Many people think the liver is the largest organ of the human body, but it's actually the skin. The skin reportedly has a surface area of 1.5–2.0 square meters. I wondered how much space mine took up. So many weight-loss surgery patients were having procedures to remove excess skin that it had become the fastest-growing field in plastic surgery.[1] I had lost weight more slowly than gastric bypass patients, so people were curious if I had gotten better results or if I looked like a melted candle anyway.

My skin had gotten looser. Skin looseness is a weird phenomenon that I suspect you have to see to understand. My body at its fattest was like a Ziploc bag filled with water. It had been squishy, but firm. If you drained half the water without letting any air in, the bag was still squishy, but it flopped around easily. That's how the loose skin was. It wasn't just skin either. Skin is only several millimeters thick at the most, like on your eyelids or between your fingers. Fat and other tissue was attached beneath it.

The way the skin looked depended on how gravity was draping it, like fabric flung across a dressmaker's mannequin. When I was standing up, it all flowed downward and looked respectable. My thighs and what I could see of my butt were getting saggy. The gut flab known as the pannus was still there, though considerably smaller than it had ever been. I could now visually confirm I had female anatomy without digging out the hand mirror.

My upper arms looked like someone cut the sleeve pattern for my skin four sizes too big. I didn't know if my breasts were less firm in comparison to other women's since I had never had the opportunity to fondle another woman's boobs. They looked remarkably perky for what they'd gone through, at least what remained of them.

The skin was most noticeable when I was doing push-ups while wearing sweatpants and a sports bra. The skin dangled toward the mat like a hammock draped from my breastbone to my pubic bone. If I were actually able to do a full push-up, I suspect my skin might have brushed the ground on the descent.

The extra skin didn't bother me. I was fascinated by it, not disgusted, as if I had grown a sixth finger. I'd seen pictures of people who had much worse skin problems than I did. I'd seen a skin-removal surgery on cable for a woman whose breasts looked like a pair of tube socks with coins at the bottom. My skin was in incredibly good condition for someone who'd lost almost two hundred pounds. I was young, I'd never smoked, and never tanned, so the skin had retained a lot of its elasticity. At my last doctor's visit my physician told me it would tighten up even more, but I didn't really believe her. I was never under any illusions that I would score the cover of the *Sports Illustrated* swimsuit edition when this was all done. I had low expectations, and they were being exceeded.

I was more concerned with function than form. My body could do so many cool things now. I could point my leg out straight from my body at a right angle. I could bend my knees up to my chest and wrap my arms around them easily. My body was awesome! I didn't mind the loose skin. I felt like I did about the Oldsmobile I'd owned that had been dented by a woman jabbering on her cell phone as she pulled out of a parking space. Her insurance company paid me $700 to get it repaired, but I just pocketed the money and kept driving the car. I thought the dent nicely distracted from the small rust stain developing near the gas tank. It still ran fine, so I didn't see any need to spend the money on an aesthetic problem.

I hadn't entirely ruled out getting plastic surgery to remove the extra skin, but I wasn't in any rush. I had read other people's accounts of their tummy tucks, which sounded more painful than a three-month stay with the Spanish Inquisition in the Iron Maiden bedroom suite. The term "tummy tuck" suggested a very simple procedure. You can easily tuck in hospital corners when you make your bed or tuck your shirt into your pants. If I had a tummy tuck, it would be weeks before I was healed enough to make my bed, and my pants wouldn't fit for months because of the swelling. I would spend the first two weeks lying on the couch in pain, eating painkillers like M&M's. It would take at least another month or two before I could walk around comfortably and pick up objects off the floor, and up to six months for all the swelling to disappear. And since I wouldn't be able to exercise for months, I'd lose some of the fitness and flexibility that I so valued.

My decision would depend on what my body ended up looking like, and how much that bothered me. If it annoyed me enough, I might submit to the horrors of voluntary plastic surgery. The cost would be a factor too, as would getting that much time off work. I was leaning toward staying out of a hospital gown, even though I could tie one around my back now. Not too many people saw me naked besides my doctor, anyway. The skin didn't bother me and my physician didn't seem concerned about it. I would just have to carefully screen any other people who might see that much skin to make sure they weren't going to freak out and dump me over it. But if they did, I was better off without them anyway. The money could probably be better spent on a trip to Europe or on whatever fancy technological gadget I was coveting this month.

The loose skin was fun to play with. I wasn't sure I wanted to get rid of it. It was like warm bread dough. I would squeeze it when I was in the restroom and roll it around between my fingers. If we were blind men and women who decided what was beautiful by touch, the obese would be regarded as supermodels.

Although I was thinner now, I still had to think about food and exercise several times a day. It was part of the regular maintenance required for my body, just like combing my hair, brushing my teeth, and showering. It was something I had to do, lest I be the crazy, smelly girl with fuzzy white teeth and a beer belly. Someone left a comment on the blog saying I was obsessed with dieting and weight loss, but that was like accusing me of being obsessed with going to the bathroom because I had to pee five or six times a day.

The weight loss was beginning to seem incidental, anyway. I was enjoying being fit and powerful for its own sake, regardless of whether all that running was helping me fit into that snug tartan skirt I'd bought from the thrift store. So many women focused solely on the weight loss, their self-esteem wobbling with every movement of the scale. I preferred to think like an athlete, feeding my body what it needed and pushing it to its limits, and the weight loss tended to follow. I needed to do what I was doing because I loved it. I wasn't a blogger because I wanted to be a millionaire. I couldn't eat healthy and exercise only because I wanted to lose weight.

I wouldn't give up my vinyl-coated dumbbells resting next to the TV set even if I never lost another pound. I took pride in carrying a twenty-pound lamp across a retail store under my arm, much to the horror of the elderly, female cashier who rushed to offer me a cart before I'd even set the box down on her conveyor belt. The light certainly wasn't lightweight, but it wasn't as if I'd chained a nightstand

and matching vanity to my back as I traipsed down the aisles. It irked me that people assumed I was weak because I was female. Part of the reason I'd hauled the item across the store was *because* it was work. It was the same reason I parked far out in the parking lot and took the stairs. Where other people looked for ways to take exertion out of their lives, I was constantly sneaking in ways to make my body work a little harder.

I delighted in hauling a tub of kitty litter up the creaky wooden steps to my apartment. It weighed twenty-seven pounds, which at the time was exactly one pound less than the distance to my goal. When I first began dropping weight, I measured how many pounds I'd lost in terms of kitty litter tubs to get a sense of how heavy I'd been. One tub became two became three until the numbers went so high I stopped being able to convert weight to tubs anymore. Now the kitty litter was relevant again because I could carry the amount of weight I had to lose.

I'd come so far, but I was always learning something new. I was never going to graduate from weight-loss school. I was reminded of this when I bought new running shoes. My old pair had worn through the inner lining of the heel. This had happened before, but I assumed my feet were deformed and misshapen and narrow in the heel. As I was tying my new shoes, I decided to lace them up all the way to the top instead of stopping on the second-to-last hole as I usually did. I'd never laced my shoes up all the way because that made them too tight. I preferred them loose so I could slip my feet into them in the mornings without having to untie and retie the laces.

Yes, I was too lazy to tie my shoes. Take it as proof that even lazy people can lose weight.

After lacing my shoes up, I went running. My shoes were clinging tightly to the back of my feet instead of rubbing loosely against them as they had always done before. They fit so much better; it was amazing. I also felt amazingly stupid when I realized I had traveled hundreds of miles in improperly laced footwear. Too bad the conflict in the Middle East wasn't as easy a problem to solve. I could only hope that another two years from now I didn't discover I'd been doing something equally foolish like drinking water from the wrong side of the cup, at least when I wasn't trying to get rid of the hiccups.

Even if I didn't know how to tie my shoelaces, the confidence I'd gained from conquering so many obstacles was spreading into other areas of my life. Near the end of winter when I walked to my car one night after work, I noticed the front passenger tire was somewhat deflated. I inspected the rim and noticed a dent. I needed the spare tire, and not the one around my waist, though that one was pretty deflated too. I lifted the trunk and started unscrewing the lid to the tire compartment. I paused. I could just call up to my office and get one of the guys I worked with to help me. I considered the option for twenty seconds before mumbling, "Screw that. I can change my own damned tire." It was light out, and I was in a safe area, so there wasn't any reason not to.

I spent the next thirty minutes figuring out how to work a jack and forcing the lug nuts to let go of their clinging emotional need to stay attached to my tire. I leaned my entire body weight onto the wrench to gain leverage, somewhat lamenting that I was lighter than I used to be. Ultimately the nuts were no match for my new muscles. I prevailed and attached the spare tire.

At which time I discovered the spare was kind of flat too.

I figured it didn't matter which deflated tire I rode home on. I got out of there and inflated the tire at a gas station later. Kneeling on cold concrete, squatting down to check the position of the jack, forcing those damned lug nuts off—all that would have exhausted me two years ago.

Now I just muddled through it without much physical stress at all, though I had small bruises on my knees for days afterward.

I felt like I could conquer anything, fat or flats. Now that I was basically thin, I'd have to start looking for a new goal. I could be so much more than the girl who lost all that weight. Now that I'd lost the weight, I felt I could do anything.

CHAPTER 17

The Secret

Twelve pairs of eyes focused on me from around the circle. They were waiting to hear my expert opinion.

I was at the focus group I'd been invited to a week earlier by a college girl trying to score an A on her final project. Her team wanted to brainstorm ideas about how to reduce obesity in central Indiana so they could create an educational campaign for their visual communications class. I'd always secretly liked the fact that there was an obesity epidemic; it made me feel less alone and less to blame if there were millions of other people with the same problem.

The only problem now was I had no idea how to reduce obesity in central Indiana.

My best idea was to snatch fat people off the street, bind them up in the back of an unmarked van, and dump them in Ohio. If we took away their cell phones and identification they would be stranded in the Buckeye state and Indiana's problem would be solved. This strategy worked pretty well for the trapper who had caught a raccoon in our crawl space and relocated it to another county.

These people seemed to think I was a weight-loss expert. They sure had been happy to see someone attend their meeting who wasn't related to them. Their faces had been so eager when they greeted me at the door, as if they were surprised I'd actually come inside instead of turning around in the driveway and making a quick getaway.

"Well, I read that if you make stairwells prettier by painting them and putting up nice art, people will be more inclined to use them," I said. "And if people are allowed to wear casual clothes to work, they'll move around more. Who wants to hike up four flights of stairs in high heels, right?"

The long-haired blond in a lavender sweater running the video camera nodded in agreement. "That's a good idea," she said.

Whew. I had them fooled. Those ideas surely sounded better than my plot to sabotage the city's elevators.

The short brunette leading the meeting spoke up. "Moving on to the next topic, do you think there are stereotypes about the obese and if so, what are they?"

I bit into the celery stick I'd snatched off the self-consciously healthy snack table. It would have been rather hypocritical to be serving cookies and chips at the obesity focus group. Carol, the overweight, middle-aged woman sitting next to me, started to speak. I assumed she was a mother of one of the group's members.

"Well, I've gained some weight in the past couple of years," she said softly as her blue eyes carefully studied the workmanship of the hardwood floors. "And I can't say I really like it. I hope people don't think I'm lazy. I've just got a busy life, and it's hard to find the time to eat right and exercise."

She seemed conflicted. I was still getting used to my new identity as the thin girl, while she was adjusting to her new identity as the fat woman. She might have stereotypes about fat people that now conflicted with her self-image. It was hard for me to imagine a time when I hadn't been fat. Did this woman remember a time when she hadn't been thin?

"It's hard," I told her, trying to be reassuring.

The proctor decided to jump in. "Carol, you missed the introductions since you came in late, but Jennette has lost over half her body weight."

Carol's eyebrows lifted in surprise.

"Wow, that's impressive!" she said. I felt as if weight loss were now considered a skill I possessed. Check out Jennette, she can wiggle her pinkie toe and lose massive amounts of weight! Too bad it wasn't a very handy skill. I could make myself thinner, but despite what this group thought, I didn't really know how to make anyone else skinnier. I couldn't possess people's bodies and force them to eat healthy diets and exercise. If I had a practical skill, like woodworking, at least I could make my friends some spice racks.

"So, can I ask you something?" Carol asked. My hands tensed around my diet soda, and I started to feel anxious as I guessed what was coming next.

"What's your secret?"

Everyone wanted to know the secret. It was as if I were one of a dozen people on the planet who knew the undisclosed blend of herbs and spices used in Kentucky Fried Chicken. Here's the secret: If you take the second letter of every third word on the bottom of every page in this book, reverse it, and then translate it from Portuguese to English, the magical secret to weight loss will be revealed to you. Once you have wasted an hour of your time trying to find this quick and easy answer, you'll figure out the real secret. There *is* no secret.

Weight loss was a personal decision requiring a lot of commitment and work, as serious as deciding to get married or moving to another city for a new job. Sometimes I felt as if I'd married my body and spent the last two years going through couples counseling working out our problems.

"Oh, I've been following a diet and exercising a lot," I said, taking a sip of my soda.

"I wish I had as much willpower as you," she replied.

"Willpower's overrated," I said before I burped. "Excuse me."

Willpower was the ability to fight against intrinsic human nature. It could work for brief spurts, but it was a stopgap, sandbags built against a rising river that would eventually burst through the temporary dam, not a permanent solution. You could use willpower to hold your bladder on a long bus trip, but eventually you'd reach a point where you pissed your pants. You could try to stop eating, but it was an essential human behavior. Eventually your body's will to survive would overthrow any willpower you had to stop eating.

I would often read blogs of people failing in their weight-loss efforts who lamented their lack of willpower, as if their wills were being run by a half-dead AAA battery. I doubted willpower was typically the problem. They'd just been trained to blame themselves for being fat, as if it were a personality flaw. If you were motivated enough to start a weight-loss blog and attempt a dieting plan, you at least had some willpower.

They spent a lot of time blaming their failures on lack of inner strength, when I suspected it had more to do with an environment that made it difficult to incorporate exercise or good foods into their lives, or perhaps ignorance about what a healthy diet and proper exercise were. It was such a waste of time to blame themselves when they should have been trying to figure out what the real problem was.

The population was getting fatter and fatter. I didn't think it was because there had been a sudden drain on the country's willpower. Our world was making it easier to become a fat person. If you didn't actively adjust your environment and habits to account for that, you could end up getting fat, no deep-seated psychological issues with food required.

Willpower was good for getting me to speed up my grocery cart as I passed the Oreos strategically placed next to the milk section. It was good for making me avoid eye contact with the Girl Scouts selling cookies outside the grocery store. But using willpower as the energy source for a long-term weight-loss plan was like trying to power an aircraft carrier with a hamster running in a wheel.

Carol wasn't deterred. "What diet are you on?" she asked. I didn't want to tell her. I didn't want to make her believe there was one magical cure-all diet. I didn't want her to try it and fail and think she was doomed to being fat forever. Occasionally someone would email me after reading my blog and ask what my typical daily food plan was. People seemed to think that if they ate the exact same foods as I did, they would become thin too. Maybe they would, but I found it important that I actually *liked* everything I ate. I doubted another person on the planet would like exactly the same foods I did, just as it was unlikely that someone would like every single MP3 in my music collection. Asking what diet I was on was like asking Yo-Yo Ma what kind of cello he played and then expecting to buy one and become a brilliant cellist. A good instrument was helpful, but you needed to know how to play it. I wasn't a nutritionist, and I had no desire to become one, so I couldn't prescribe meal plans for every person I met. Eating healthy was important, but people focused so much on food that they forgot it was equally important to find something that fit into their own lives. Maybe my reticence was the reason people thought I had a secret that I wouldn't tell them. In reality, everything I learned was available in library books or online.

But Carol seemed interested, and I felt the pressure of all those eyes searching me for answers that I didn't necessarily have. I told her what diet I was following and hoped I wasn't leading her astray. I still felt like a dork whenever I uttered the word "carb."

"Are you exercising too?" she asked.

"Yeah, some running and Pilates. It helps me de-stress," I told her.

She sighed, "Yeah, stress is a problem for me. I tend to go for salty snacks when I'm anxious or feeling depressed."

Carol's daughter was sitting next to her and piped up. "I've been telling her maybe she should see a therapist to talk about the emotional eating stuff. I think it's only when we work through all the reasons that we overeat that we can get thin," she said.

I didn't remember working through any emotional issues. I'd sorted out a lot of thoughts on my blog, but I didn't recall having any major breakthroughs. But I'd also read journals by women who were brought to tears after they ate an entire package of chocolate donuts, including the crumbs left in the folds of their T-shirts. Some women told tales of overbearing mothers who nagged them constantly about how fat their size-8 asses were and put them on strict diets. I guessed emotional eating was more of an issue for some people than others. It was possible I'd had a breakthrough and didn't even realize it.

"If she did it, so can you, Mom," her daughter said as she reached over to squeeze her mom's hand.

I restrained myself from rolling my eyes and sighing. I hated it when people said that. I did believe that everyone could lose weight, but my personal success neither increased nor decreased their chances of doing so. When someone won the lottery, it neither increased nor decreased my chances of winning the jackpot next week. People could lose weight because it was physically possible, not because of anything I had done. I think Carol's daughter really meant to say, "Look, it's not impossible!" Keeping it off was far more difficult than losing it. In one obesity study, subjects were fed a specific number of calories for several months in controlled conditions.[1] Everyone lost weight, though some people's metabolisms slowed down to compensate for the lack of food. It was when you were let out of the lab that you ran into problems.

It was unfair to tell someone it was possible to lose weight simply because I had done it. I had a lot of advantages; I was a single woman without any kids and a low-stress job that required only forty hours of work a week. I was the star of "The Me Show," starring, written by, and produced by me. The only other life form I was responsible for taking care of was my cat. I could lead a pretty selfish life.

I could easily find the time to cook and exercise. I was doing okay financially after I'd paid off all my credit cards and my gallbladder surgery. I could spend money on fitness equipment and kickboxing class and fresh produce. I had never yo-yo dieted, so I wasn't mentally exhausted by the idea of watching what I ate. I also hadn't experienced any major life changes in the past two years. My move had been only across town, not to another state or country. Everyone I loved had been kind enough to stay alive, so I could stay focused on my weight-loss goals. Honestly, my life was kind of boring, and as far as weight loss was concerned, that was a boon. I got religion about my new lifestyle and had the time and resources to pursue it.

I didn't know much about Carol's life, but I doubted hers was similar to mine. She probably had to cook for her high school–age daughter. If she had a husband, she might be cooking for him as well and eating larger portions in an effort to keep up with him at the dinner table. Her job could be stressful, which might lead her to snack on candy bars from the vending machine. I didn't know if she lived in a neighborhood with sidewalks where it would be safe to walk or if she could afford a gym membership to go exercise. If anything were out of control in her life or unsatisfying, she might search for comfort and control by indulging in tasty foods. If money were tight, a bag of potato chips would always be cheaper than a bag of apples. I'd never seen someone double-coupon a pound of pears.

The stupidest things had sometimes kept me from overeating. If my cat curled up on my lap while I was watching TV, I wouldn't get up for that second fudge pop because I couldn't bring myself to interrupt his mewing. When I served my meal on smaller plates, it looked bigger and stopped me from eating bigger portions. When I started walking on the trail, I headed for thirty minutes in each direction instead of the total fifty minutes I had done on the treadmill because the math was easier to figure out on my watch.

None of this meant Carol couldn't lose weight. It just meant it was harder for some people than others. I had friends who could eat a bucket of lard and still didn't seem to gain a pound. They would only gain twenty bucks, because I bet them they wouldn't eat a bucket of lard. Disadvantages weren't an excuse, just an explanation. "Because it's hard" wasn't a good reason not to at least *try* to do something. It was important to pave the path of least resistance, to make it as easy as possible for you to live a healthy lifestyle.

We could sit in this discussion group all day and throw theories at one another. No one thing had made me fat, and no one thing had made me thin. It was a complex, intricate set of variables and circumstances. It was an advanced equation that I had to figure out how to balance. Everyone got her own math problem to solve: some from the introduction to algebra course, others from advanced calculus.

Starting seemed to be the hardest part. Getting my body to lose weight had been like trying to start a car that would have preferred to spend retirement rusting in a parking spot in the shade of an elm tree. I had to turn and turn the key, pop the clutch, give it more gas, until for some reason it magically kicked into life. I didn't ask why; I just got it in gear and kept going before it could die again.

"How do you stay motivated?" Carol asked.

I should have just told her to screw motivation. If I waited for motivation to do the dishes, I'd have plates stacked on my counter so high that I couldn't open the microwave. Which I currently did. I was never motivated to do my dishes. Yet I turned on the faucet and poured out some dish soap anyway. It wasn't because I wanted to have fun with bubbles; it was because I had to. I couldn't bring myself to eat off paper plates.

I'd read other people's weight-loss stories in magazines and there was always a point in the story where they had a huge revelation that kicked them in the fat pants. They couldn't fit in the roller-coaster harness or their uncle died from heart disease. But why wait until you'd wasted forty bucks on an amusement park ticket or you were buying huge black pants for a funeral? I thought I'd had my moment when I had gallbladder surgery, but I spent more than a year after that just as fat as I ever was. People waited for motivation to find them, but they needed to go out and find motivation. It's doubtful that you would get to the bottom of that pint of ice cream and find the message "You need to lose weight" written on the bottom.

This was all easier said than done, of course. It's hard to get unstuck, but it takes even longer to pull your feet out of the gum left on the sidewalk if you wait for someone else to come along with Goo Gone. You just have to do it, even though you don't want to. If you saw diet and exercise as optional, you were screwed. It was nonnegotiable.

"Oh, I don't know. It helps if you find exercise that you like to do."

Carol nodded her head. "Well, I hope I can do it too. I don't like being so fat."

"Oh Mom, you're not fat," her daughter said.

Well, actually she was, I thought. The problem wasn't that Carol was fat, it was that "fat" was considered a dirty word. It had become an insult when really it was just a description of how someone looked. It wasn't any different from saying someone was tall or short, blond or brunette. Maybe if we weren't so afraid to use the word we could stop seeing it as such a bad thing to be. Yet it seemed impossible to use the word "fat" without sending an emotional charge.

"You've just been making some bad food choices lately," her daughter said.

I was making a lot of choices these days. I would always go for the slice of whole-wheat over the white bread. Sweet potatoes would beat normal potatoes in all my vegetable wrestling matches. I peeled the skin off the chicken even if that made me a poultry scalper. All those little choices in the day added up to something bigger. It was like stacking every brick to make a glorious cathedral or sitting at a loom every day, weaving thread in and out to make a glittering tapestry. Losing weight required a lot of constant thinking and decision making.

I had certainly chosen to become thinner, but my fatness was more a result of the choices I *hadn't* been making. I had woken up that morning and come to this meeting. I did not go to Bermuda. Had I *chosen* not to go to Bermuda? In all the time I spent picking out camouflage socks that matched my green top, measuring the proper amount of water into my instant oatmeal, and locking the door as I left, not once did a thought bubble appear over my head saying, "Hey, I could go to Bermuda!" This was partly because I was not a cartoon character and partly because the thought never occurred to me. If I never even saw this as an option, it wasn't fair to say I made a choice not to go to Bermuda.

Similarly, when I was fat I had never hit a situation in my daily routine when I had to consider "Do I get fat or do I stay thin?" I didn't live on the *Let's Make a Deal* set with Curtain Number One or Two to choose from. At the most, I encountered situations in which I had to choose between two options that would lead me to either of the possible end points of thinness and fatness.

The problem was I didn't know some of the choices I was making were going to make me as fat as I became. I knew Twinkies weren't a health food, but I had no idea exactly how bad they were for me. If there had been a moment that morning when I had considered going to Bermuda instead of the meeting, I would have also had to consider that such a choice would probably get me fired when I didn't show up for work the next week. It would also drain my savings account, which I'd worked hard to bulk up. If I had flown off anyway and then discovered I'd upset my family by missing our planned dinner party, would I have chosen to alienate them?

Similarly, I wasn't choosing to be fat when I knew little about nutrition and exercise, when I had no concept of how many calories I was taking in every day and didn't even know how many calories I *should* be taking in. I was still personally responsible for my actions, actions that led me to obesity, but I was ignorant or at least partially ignorant, which prevented me from making a conscious choice to be fat. The word "choice" implied intent, which I lacked. I was like a driver who rear-ended the car in front of me while fiddling with the radio station—I was responsible for the accident, but I hadn't chosen to hit someone. I'd chosen to take my eyes off the road and had paid the price.

I spent one summer in high school at an academic camp where I ate pizza almost every day for lunch. I also had a not-so-secret affair with the soft-serve ice cream, and I wasn't the only one, that whore. While I knew the ice cream was a bad idea, it never occurred to me that eating that much pizza was going to keep me fat too. I don't know how I made it past admissions with this blatant stupidity. I was personally responsible for my food choices, but I wouldn't say I was choosing to be fat when I chose pizza. I was just a nutritional idiot who didn't realize the full repercussions of my actions. If the dozens of people I saw at the McDonald's drive-through every evening truly knew how much a Big Mac cost them in terms of energy input and output, half of them would probably squeal their tires for the closest Subway. They might even get out and jog there to burn off the extra calories from that morning's Egg McMuffin.

Having options was another factor in choice. Some people had lives that were more predisposed to make them fat. If you had decided to eat healthy, what did you do when the cafeteria had only donuts or danishes left for breakfast? How easy was it for you to exercise if you lived in an urban environment? Is it really a choice not to go to the gym if you can't afford a membership?

Saying that fat people choose to be fat is at the very least oversimplifying matters, and at the most, it implies we have more control over our lives than we actually do. Not everything that happens to you is a direct result of a choice you made. If it were, we'd all be all-powerful and all-knowing. If an idiot rear-ends your car, it isn't your fault simply because you chose to go for a drive. Some things happen to us that we have no control over. Choices we make sometimes have consequences that we are unaware of when we make our decisions.

That's not to say we have no control, either. Fat people can get thinner. I still had the fat pants to prove it. I made different choices and altered my behavior, and now I had seen the rewards. But a lot of my success came from awakening to the fact that I *hadn't* been making choices. I wasn't debating "Should I run tonight or not?" The thought never occurred to me. I didn't know that eating a big bowl of macaroni and cheese would leave me tired. I never considered eating something better. However, I did know that eating a jar of frosting with a spoon wasn't making me the next Kate Bosworth either. That one was all on me. It was the difference between accidental manslaughter and premeditated homicide.

I chose the actions that ultimately made me fat, but I wasn't always aware that the food I was eating had so many calories, and I didn't always have a treadmill in my bedroom. I was responsible for being fat, but it wasn't always a choice.

I had no idea how to tell Carol this, though. I finished chomping on my celery stick and the discussion concluded. Sadly, we did not solve the obesity epidemic of central Indiana that afternoon. I got up to get my jacket from the hat stand. Carol came over to see me off and said, "Congratulations again. You seem really happy."

I was happier, but it wasn't just because I was thin. I had changed a lot on the outside, but only because I'd changed so much on the inside. People saw this brightness in me and assumed it was because I was skinnier.

"You don't look like you need to lose any more weight, either," she added. There's a sentence I'd never thought I'd hear someone say to me.

"Thanks," I said as I opened the door. "And good luck." I shut the door softly between us.

A couple of weeks later it was warm enough to go outside without a jacket, so I headed straight for the trail. It was odd to think I was excited to go outside. I'd always hated the outdoors growing up. In fifth grade, I'd hid under a table so I wouldn't have to go out to play kickball. I'm sure the class's pet guinea pig was happy to have the company or at least happy to be tormented by one fifth-grader instead of thirty. I laced up my shoes tightly, headed for the gate, and started walking to warm up my muscles. I passed a woman with an amazing physique. Thankfully I'd stopped playing "Is she fatter than me?" lately and had started playing "How many reps will make me that ripped?"

I picked up my pace and broke into a slow run. The rasp of air rushing through my nasal passages sounded like intermittent static on the TV, sparking off and on while someone adjusted the antenna. I was now able to complete an eleven-minute mile, but I knew my pace wouldn't break any land-speed records or even beat the eight-year-old on training wheels ahead of me. I didn't care.

I felt breeze on the back of my sweaty neck and was hit with a sudden blast of joy. Even though I didn't have a boyfriend, and I didn't have a million dollars, and my toilet was probably in the process of breaking, I was experiencing these unexpected hits of happiness more and more lately. I was closer to joy now than ever before, as if I had moved next door to it and caught glimpses of it mowing its lawn and getting the mail from time to time.

The sun was burning hydrogen and helium to create dazzling light that sparkled off the water below the bridge. The hot and cold air collided to form a breeze that brushed my hair back in the wind. As I inhaled for two steps, exhaled for one, I felt the rhythm of my running flowing through me like the air in my lungs. Ryan Adams was singing in my ears telling me I was so alive, so alive. I couldn't disagree.

If there were a secret, this was it.

CHAPTER 18

Killing the Fat Girl

So, that's the end, right? I got thin and now I get to live happily ever after. I'll never step foot in the plus-size section of another department store. I'll eat sugar-free gelatin desserts for the rest of my life. Someday I'll meet the perfect man, and we'll laugh at my fat pictures and joke about how ridiculous it is that I ever looked like that. Let's close the book on this fairy-tale story, put it on the shelf, and knock back some champagne with my fairy godmother.

Too bad I could still get fat again.

It happens. A lot.[1] If the diet industry knew how to successfully help people maintain long-term weight loss, it would have put itself out of business decades ago. People like me have a fat chance of staying thin. I'm going to roll the dice anyway and gamble that I can maintain my weight. It's better to play the game even though I might lose than to sit it out entirely.

I'm on permanent probation. I'll be making weekly check-ins with my parole officer forever. His office is my bathroom floor and his face displays three numbers. He lets me walk all over him. If I stop exercising and stop eating right, I *will* go back to fat prison. There is no leniency.

I have to think about food and exercise more than I'd like to, but that's the price I pay, and it will probably never go away.

My metabolism will slow down as I age and ten or twenty pounds might start to creep back on. There are weeks now when the numbers start to climb back up, and I worry that I might have to dig out a larger pair of jeans. I don't have a box of skinny clothes at the bottom of the closet any more, just a box labeled FAT CLOTHES (IN CASE OF EMERGENCY).

I don't think I'm going to get fat again, but who ever plans to gain back the weight? No one plans a car accident, either. When things are going well it's difficult to remember how hard life was before. But to gain back all two hundred-and-something pounds, I would have to completely stop caring. I can't unlearn everything I've learned. I think my chances are good for success because I've accepted the fact that my body needs constant care and attention. I haven't been cured of obesity, I'm just in remission. There is no fat vaccine. I have realistic goals and I won't be heartbroken if I never wear a size 4 dress.

The funny thing is, that fat girl hiding in my mother's photo albums, the one in the ugly clothes with the slumped shoulders, she had a pretty good life. She had a cat who curled up on her soft, fleshy belly for naps. She had a family with a sense of humor, who never made her feel bad about herself. She got good grades and was frequently the teacher's pet. She always had a safe place to sleep, food to eat, and a place to call home. Given the choice between that life and the life of a skinny starlet in rehab, I'd put the fat suit back on fast enough to jam the zipper.

Many thin people would be surprised that fat people could feel that way about themselves. A survey done by the Rudd Center for Food Policy and Obesity showed that nearly half of the people questioned would rather give up a year of their lives than be obese.[2]

Between 15 and 30 percent would rather get divorced, become infertile, be depressed, or become alcoholic. People are scared of fat. Fear can sometimes be a good thing. Fear means the bad thing hasn't happened yet. But sometimes, you experience the worst possible thing you can imagine and surprisingly discover it is survivable. All the panicking and freaking out over fat is worse than any love handle. Fearing that I could become fat again is a waste of time. I would never have consciously chosen to become morbidly obese, just as I would never fling myself into the path of a speeding Volkswagen. We don't get to choose the obstacles life sets in our path, yet there is a lot to be learned from jumping those hurdles.

Obesity gave me a great sense of perspective. I don't have any unrealistic expectations about how thin any woman should be. I look at magazine covers in the grocery store aisle and feel genuinely sad for the emaciated superstars who are picked on for being anorexic twigs or gluttonous pigs. I see women who probably wear size 12 jeans and think they look thin. I can appreciate being thinner more than someone who has never been fat ever could.

Obesity also made me understand that the package you come in affects the way people treat you. Being fat was like having a built-in asshole detector. People who were jerks didn't go out of their way to be nice to me. It must be hard if you've always been thin and you've always seen the best sides of people at first. How can you determine who the jerks are if they come at you wearing disguises? I've certainly never had to wonder if I got anywhere because of my looks.

But when I talk to unhappy fat friends, I sometimes feel as though I have moved into a different class, like I'm a poor little match girl who now owns a lighter fluid company. I wish I could tell them how to get to the happy place where I am, but the route doesn't seem to be found in any road atlas. If it did, I'd make photocopies for everyone and circle the destination in a big, yellow highlighter and tie balloons to the mailbox so you could all join the party. But I can't. You have to find it yourself without the aid of a global positioning device. You don't necessarily have to be thin to come inside, either.

I do love being thin, though I still carry enough weight that some people might consider me chubby. When I'm walking through the mall I occasionally have to remind myself that I can shop in the normal stores. Sometimes I walk into the department store and try on dresses that cost more than my cable and electric bills combined just to see how cute I look in them. But I usually put those frocks back on the rack because I prefer to be able to continue using my hair dryer and checking my email. Every time I look in the mirror I still think, "I look so freaking hot." Sometimes I think I would look even hotter if I lost ten more pounds.

One friend said I smile more now. Another said I was glowing. I *am* a lot happier. I think people assume it's because I'm thin. That's only part of it. At the beginning I saw weight loss as the ultimate goal, but once I started taking care of myself I started living a life that made me happier, which also happened to make me thinner. It's easy to confuse the two. I've heard it said that people need to love themselves no matter what, but I think you have to earn your own love through the things you do for yourself. I had to shape myself into someone worth loving, someone worthy of my own respect.

I've changed so much through this experience that I wonder if I should add an upgrade number to my name to alert people to all my new features. Introducing Jennette 2.0, now with less fat and a more huggable interface. Last week I walked down the trail to an organic grocery store to buy pears and found myself wondering, *If I've been replaced by a pod person, would I know about it?* I've heard a rumor that every cell in your body replaces itself at least once in the course of seven years. Sometimes I wonder if my data got slightly corrupted and now I'm a copy of someone I never was. I might just be growing up.

I probably don't even notice some of the ways I've changed. I can't stand outside of myself and observe my actions like both the rat and the laboratory scientist. I always liked who I was, but maybe people can just see that better now. When I hear my voice on an answering machine I think, *That cannot possibly be me. I do not sound like that.* But I do. Perhaps the image I am projecting now more closely matches the image I had of myself all along.

I cooked dinner for my mother when she visited my apartment a couple of months ago. I coated some chicken breasts in Italian dressing and sautéed them while green beans seasoned with garlic cooked in the microwave and I brought some water to boil on the back burner for couscous. She stared at me and shook her head.

"Who would have ever thought," she murmured.

"What?" I said.

"My daughter, the culinary genius."

"I could throw in a cartwheel to really impress you, but I have to flip the chicken now," I replied.

When she left, she wrapped her arms far enough around me to grab her own elbows, squeezing me tight in her embrace.

When I began this journey, I thought I would get to the finish line and write a tirade about everyone who discriminated against me, saying I was the same person thin as I was fat. Only that isn't true. I can cook. I can run for miles. I feel proud and powerful. I accomplished a huge task and took control of my life. I feel like I'm driving now, not just sitting in the back seat of a stinky taxicab with a questionable upholstery stain. I'm more myself. I have the amplifier turned up to eleven.

I live a life with less fear. I'm not afraid I'll have to ask the stewardess for a seat belt extender on the plane. I'm not afraid to walk into a clothing store and be able to buy only a pair of socks. I don't fear looking at the photos from my brother's wedding, when I proudly wore a sleeveless dress to show off my new arm muscles. I didn't make it to goal by then as I planned, but I felt beautiful and alive, and I broke my dress strap as I kicked my heels up to "Shout."

I don't have to feel the pain of obesity anymore and not just in my aching knees. When I ride the bus, I'm not the fat lady whom everyone avoids sitting next to. I remember avoiding eye contact as people swiped their bus passes. I remember praying no one would be left on his or her feet because I was too fat to sit next to. But remembering a feeling isn't the same as hearing your heart quicken in fear and feeling ashamed that your thighs are spilling into the next seat. I've gotten off that bus and all I have left is a ticket stub to remember the ride.

The world is a more hopeful place now, as though the magnetic poles switched and I'm living on the positive end of the planet instead of the negative end. Anything seems possible. I am, after all, the girl who lost more than two hundred pounds. I'm not entirely convinced that if I stepped out my second-story bedroom window and decided I could hang glide on my batwings of arm flesh, that I would land in the bushes and break my leg. And if I did end up in a full body cast, at least I tried to fly. There's nothing to be ashamed of when you fail to do something great. When you go out on a limb, sometimes you fly and sometimes the limb breaks. Even if you end up lying on your back with branches poking your butt cheeks, at least you have a great view of the stars.

A lot of people have called me an inspiration. It's odd being a success story, to be the girl who has something so many other people want. I always had a sweet tooth, but I was never a fan of the sugary, sweet stories about people overcoming adversity. They always seemed fake, built up by the author to tell a good story while quietly brushing the bad stuff under the carpet to be ignored. But I think I was just afraid that they were true, that there were people who loved their lives and had sunshine coming out of their asses and that I would never be one of them. I suppose I'm one of those annoying bastards now. I don't have any light shining out of my rectum, though. I'm bendy enough now that I checked. I've achieved something many people want to accomplish, but it doesn't make me any more special or amazing than anyone else. I don't think people give themselves enough credit. We're all capable of a lot more than we think.

Sometimes I feel I need to apologize for being so happy, to say I'm sorry to all the people who want to be thin but are stuck being fat. When I shine so bright, I'm bound to deepen the shadows in their lives. But my life isn't perfect either. Being thin hasn't solved all my problems, and the problems I do have can no longer be blamed on my obesity. Overweight women who read my blog frequently ask if people treat me better now, as if no one would ever be mean to me again because I'm thin. I get cut off in traffic by insecure men driving SUVs even though I'm thin. I had to wait in line at the DMV to finally renew my driver's license and replace my fat photo even though I'm thin. I have not been seduced by a hot Latino lover over a latte at the bookstore even though I'm thin. The grass always looks greener where the thin people live, but there are patches of crabgrass and poison ivy here too. I haven't been invited to any secret glamorous thin parties where we stand around not eating hors d'oeuvres.

In all the preceding chapters in this book you'll notice I never did meet the perfect man and run off into the sunset. There aren't any wacky dating stories either because I don't have many to tell. The longest relationship I've had with a male is with my cat, and he doesn't even have balls. But any intimacy issues I have are because of me, not because of my fat. They always were. I might be able to pick up more guys in bars now, but I have to go to the bars for that to happen. I can't expect to find new friends and lovers hiding under my couch. I got LASIK and I lost the weight, so I'm no longer a blind, fat homebody, just a seeing, thin homebody. The house of me is in a lot better shape, but it could still use some work. Construction will never be completely finished, but I could start inviting more people over.

Sometimes I joke about my old fat self and wonder if that's okay. If I were still almost four hundred pounds, I'd have to sit on someone who insulted me. I get a pass to make fun of myself, but if anyone else makes fun of the old fat girl, I feel my fists curling at my sides. She might no longer physically exist, but she's rented a back room in my mind. I don't know if I can ever evict her.

It's possible I've forgotten exactly how painful it was being fat or how hard it was to transition into a healthier lifestyle. Time might scrub my memories like steel wool scraping against a dirty pan until only the shiny spots remain. I don't know what percentage of my life I actually remember. All the time I've spent driving to and from work or brushing my teeth and showering has most likely been saved and overwritten a million times. I'm definitely grateful for all I can do now. Sometimes I squat down to pick up cat toys simply because I'm amazed that I can do so. Then I pop back up without the aid of a coffee table. I can put my foot on the bathroom counter and cut my toenails with ease. I didn't know my body was capable of such things. It's like when I discovered my cell phone could not only make calls but also play pinball games and keep a date book. I now come with extra features.

Maybe joking around is the only way I'm able to acknowledge how bad my situation was, something I couldn't do when I was living it. Distance brings perspective. I don't want to treat the old fat girl too harshly, though. My humor is self-deprecating because I don't take myself that seriously, not because I want to rip myself down.

There *is* a temptation to kill the fat girl I once was, to stab her in the neck and bury her in the azaleas. But I think she's immortal. I can run her over with my car, drown her in the toilet, asphyxiate her with a yoga strap, but she can't ever really die. She may give out a death rattle, lie limp on the floor, but she's just faking for my benefit. The fat girl will always be a part of who I am. I can't unmake myself by becoming thin.

I used to think weight loss was retroactive. If I became thin I could erase the time in my life when I was fat. All my old photos would morph to show a skinny girl smiling proud. If she didn't exist in the present, all the pain of the past would disappear. All the opportunities she missed would be lined up in front of me, so now I could go to the prom or wear a bathing suit to birthday pool parties. But it doesn't work like that. I don't get a do-over. I can have plastic surgery to remove this loose skin and sell all my fat clothes on eBay. I can move to an apartment complex where no one knows I was obese, but I will always have been the fat girl.

And that's okay. The fat girl had her issues, but she was pretty awesome too.

As I write this, I'm still about ten pounds away from my goal weight. I might have reached goal by the time you read this. Maybe not. Somewhat anticlimactic, eh? That's not how the story usually ends. There's a template for weight-loss stories: Girl gets fat, girl loses weight, girl reaches goal and rides into the sunset on a horse without breaking its back. It's like a game of Mad Libs: [Name] lost [huge number] pounds by eating [tasteless health food] and doing [painful exercise]. You could write that book yourself.

When I began this trip, my goal was a number, three digits that I hoped would appear on the digital box on my scale without having to switch the unit of weight from pounds to kilograms. But my real goal didn't have anything to do with numbers. I wanted to be happy.

I wanted to like my body. I wanted to feel comfortable in the world. All those things are true now. As long as that continues to be true, the numbers on the scale don't matter as much. They matter, just not as much.

The numbers on my scale haven't yet aligned in the manner I aimed for, but I have reached my goal. It didn't happen suddenly but sneaked up on me like my cat, sitting quietly at my feet until the moment I looked down and saw him staring into my eyes. It was like waking up from a long car trip as a child after being nestled in the back seat and wrapped in the white noise of the highway, awakening to turn my sleepy eyes out the car window and seeing our back door reflecting the porch light, wondering, *When did we get home?*

There is some fear in writing the preceding thousands of words and holding myself up as a gleaming beacon of weight-loss success, of saying, "Look how healthy and happy I am! Aren't I great?" It is like balancing on the top of a pedestal as I wave to you all, waiting for it to be kicked out from beneath me. I hope I don't wobble and break my nose on the linoleum floor. I don't know what my life will be like next year or in five years or in twenty years. None of us do. Someone I love could die and I might seek solace in tubs of ice cream. I could get married and have kids and find no time for exercise other than picking up toys. I could simply become blasé about the whole process for no reason at all and say, "Screw it!" before pitching my Pilates mat to Goodwill.

But I will fight harder than I do in any kickboxing class to stop those things from happening.

I will always have to monitor my weight. I will always have to make decisions about what I eat until the day they stop making food. There will always be days when the couch and a pair of slippers look more appealing than the trail and my dirty running shoes.

I may have lost the weight, but it could still find me again. I can try to shake it off my tail, run a red light, or careen over the railroad tracks right before the train passes by. But I can always see it in my rearview mirror a couple of car lengths behind me. I have to keep moving, weaving through traffic, or it will catch up with me again. I have to keep the gas tank full.

There's never an ending to this story. There's never a final page. There's just a point where you stop writing.

NOTES

CHAPTER 1

1 I had heard that yo-yo dieting: "Weight Cycling," *National Institutes of Health*, http://win.niddk.nih.gov/publications/cycling.htm

2 Recent studies have shown: Karen Collins, "Yo-yo dieting may have a bad rap," *MSNBC.com*, 8 July 2007, http://www.msnbc.msn.com/id/19621031

3 I was under no delusions: Dirk Taubert et al., "Chocolate and Blood Pressure in Elderly Individuals with Isolated Systolic Hypertension," *JAMA* 290.8 (2003): 1029–30.

4 For several years everyone thought fat: Delroy Alexander, Jeremy Manier, and Patricia Callahan, "The Oreo, Obesity And Us: For every fad, another cookie," *The Chicago Tribune*, 23 August 2005.

CHAPTER 3

1 To qualify for the surgery. "Gastrointestinal Surgery for Severe Obesity," *National Institutes of Health*, http://win.niddk.nih.gov/publications/gastric.htm

2 Out of 16,155 cases studied: David R. Flum et al., "Early Mortality Among Medicare Beneficiaries Undergoing Bariatric Surgical Procedures." *JAMA* 294.15 (2005): 1903–08.

3 Many more suffer complications: Robert Steinbrook, "Surgery for Severe Obesity." *New England Journal of Medicine* 350.11 (2004): 1075–79.

4   This surgery is gaining popularity: Paul E. O'Brien, Wendy A. Brown, and John B. Dixon, "Obesity, weight loss and bariatric surgery," *Medical Journal of Australia* 183.6 (2005): 310–314.

5   Disappointingly, most patients: G. D. Foster et al., "What is a reasonable weight loss? Patients' expectations and evaluations of obesity treatment outcomes," *Journal of Consulting and Clinical Psychology* 65.1 (1997): 79–85.

CHAPTER 4

1   There were interesting discussions: Abigail C. Saguy, "In a moral panic over obesity," *UCLA Today,* 23 May 2006.

2   I wanted to be paid: Victoria Colliver, "Study finds obesity takes an economic toll on workers, firms," *The San Francisco Chronicle,* 24 April 2007.

3   After reading the most recent research: Gina Kolata, *Rethinking Thin,* (New York: Farrar, Straus and Giroux, 2007).

4   People struggling to get by couldn't afford: Adam Drewnowski and S. E. Specter, "Poverty and obesity: the role of energy density and energy costs," *The American Journal of Clinical Nutrition* 79.1 (2004): 6–16.

5   Some scientists speculated obesity: Julie Steenhuysen, "Too fat? Common virus may be to blame," *Reuters,* 20 August 2007.

6   In one study, girls who took a math test: Belinda Goldsmith, "Girls do badly at math when told boys better," *Reuters,* 24 May 2007.

7   Stress and lack of sleep are bad for you: "Lack of sleep may be deadly, research shows," *Reuters,* 24 September 2007.

8   The BMI was developed: Stephanie Wilson, "How Body Mass Index Works," *How Stuff Works,* http://health.howstuffworks.com/bmi4.htm

CHAPTER 5

1   I was also kind of horny: Colette Bouchez, "Better Sex: What's Weight Got to Do with It?," *WebMD,* 25 March 2005, http://www.webmd.com /sex-relationships/guide/sex-and-weight

CHAPTER 9

1   We were supposedly the first generation: Samuel H. Preston, "Deadweight? The Influence of Obesity on Longevity," *New England Journal of Medicine* 352.11 (2005):1135-37.

2   The National Bureau of Standards conducted: "Short History of Ready-Made Clothing," *National Institute of Standards and Technology Virtual Museum*, http://museum.nist.gov/exhibits/apparel/history.htm

CHAPTER 12

1   In the western corner: Rebecca Popenoe, "Ideal," *Fat: The Anthropology of an Obsession*, eds. Don Kulick and Anne Meneley (New York: Penguin Group, 2005), 10–11.

2   This was a theory that: R. B. Harris, "Role of set-point theory in regulation of body weight," *Federation of American Societies for Experimental Biology J* 4.15 (1990): 3310–18.

3   It built up my ability to persist: Po Bronson, "How Not to Talk to Your Kids: The inverse power of praise," *New York Magazine,* 19 February 2007.

4   Earlier in the year I had read a study: Brian Wansink, James E. Painter, and Yeon-Kyung Lee, "The Office Candy Dish: Proximity's Influence on Estimated and Actual Candy Consumption," *International Journal of Obesity* 30.5 (2006): 871–5.

CHAPTER 13

1   I'd also learned obese people were paid less: Damon Darlin, "Extra Weight, Higher Costs," *The New York Times,* 2 December 2006.

2   They might keep it off for a year: Traci Mann et al., "Medicare's Search for Effective Obesity Treatments: Diets Are Not the Answer," *American Psychologist* 62.3 (2007): 220–33.

CHAPTER 14

1   When I read an article: "Teacher for $1 allegedly let kids skip gym a day," Associated Press, 16 February 2006.

CHAPTER 15

1   I had read that people became increasingly worse: Brian Wansink and Pierre Chandon, "Meal Size, Not Body Size, Explains Errors in Estimating the Calorie Content of Meals," *Ann Intern Med* 145.5 (2006): 326–32.

2   Some scientists believed that the reduced obese: R. L. Leibel and J. Hirsch, "Diminished energy requirements in reduced-obese patients," *Metabolism* 33.2 (1984):64–70.

3   Once my fat cells reached a certain threshold size: J. K. Hewitt, "The genetics of obesity: What have genetic studies told us about the environment?" *Behavior Genetics* 27.4 (1997): 353–58.

CHAPTER 16

1   So many weight-loss surgery patients: Matthew Herper, "Fastest-Growing Plastic Surgeries," *Forbes.com*, 15 May 2006, http://www.wired.com/medtech /health/news/2006/05/70889

CHAPTER 17

1   In one obesity study they locked subjects: R. L. Leibel, M. Rosenbaum, and J. Hirsch, "Changes in Energy Expenditure Resulting from Altered Body Weight," *New England Journal of Medicine* 332.10 (1995): 621–8.

CHAPTER 18

1   It happens. A lot: Suzanne Phelan et al., "Recovery from relapse among successful weight maintainers," *The American Journal of Clinical Nutrition* 78.6 (2003): 1079–84.

2   A survey done by: *Rudd Center for Food Policy and Obesity*, http://www .yale.edu/opa/newsr/06-05-16-02.all.html

ACKNOWLEDGMENTS

Thanks to all my blog readers. If you hadn't been watching my weight at the same time I was, I might never have gotten here. Thank you to all the other weight-loss bloggers for sharing your stories and letting me know I'm not alone. I would name you all, but I know I'd forget someone, so if you ever commented on my blog, just insert your name in the blank here. Thanks, _____!

Thank you to the women of BlogHer.org and especially Kalyn Denny of Kalyn's Kitchen for raving about my blog at the annual conference and hooking me up with my editor. Thank you particularly for not charging 10 percent!

Thank you to both of my editors. Brooke Warner believed in this book, helped me develop the idea, and got me started writing it. Krista Lyons-Gould gave me encouraging and insightful comments and cut out my bad jokes. Thank you both for putting up with my overactive spam filter.

Cristy Cummings Landaw has been my friend through thin and thick and thin again. Thank you for not being the least bit surprised that I wrote a book one day. I sent early drafts of the beginning chapters to Jennifer Thompson, who helped build my confidence and convince me I could figure out how to write a book after all. Cheryl Chastine took time off from studying to check for obvious medical errors. Fred Choi was my second-harshest critic after myself and this book is better because of it. Donna Martin offered her proofreading experience without being paid.

Thanks to Wendy McClure for being my book Yoda and not even making me carry her around the swamps of Dagobah on my back.

Big props to Deborah Lewis-Fravel and Christine Slaughter who helped come up with the title. Thanks to all the readers who proposed title suggestions as well.

Thank you, Dr. Maureen Morehead, my high school creative writing teacher, for teaching me about imagery.

My kitty, Officer Krupke, spent many days locked in the bedroom so I could write this book without the editorial interference of his paws on the keyboard. Kkjljdfklasjdfhlk is not a word, Krupke.

And of course, thanks to my family, who are far more important to me than losing a single pound. Thank you for loving me, fat or thin, and not screwing me up, at least not in any irreversible way.

ABOUT THE AUTHOR

Jennette Fulda was born weighing 8 pounds 5 ounces, but she eventually tipped the scales at 372 pounds before losing more than half her body weight through diet and exercise. She chronicles her weight loss journey in the popular blog *Half of Me* (pastaqueen.com), which has been reviewed in the *Wall Street Journal, Glamour,* and named a "Site We Love" by the website for Mo'Nique's F.A.T. Chance. She also contributes articles to *Capessa at Yahoo! Health* and the Condé Nast health and fitness blog *Elastic Waist.* When she is not working her ass off, she works in Indianapolis as a web developer and writer. To access exclusive bonus materials, visit www.halfassedbook.com.

BEFORE   **AFTER**

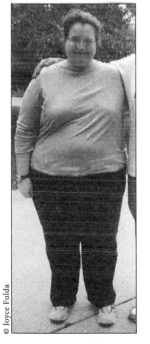

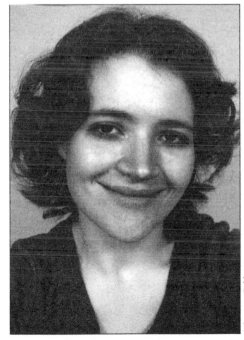

© Joyce Fulda

© Jennette Fulda

SELECTED TITLES FROM SEAL PRESS

For more than thirty years, Seal Press has published groundbreaking books.
By women. For women. Visit our website at www.sealpress.com.
Check out the Seal Press blog at www.sealpress.com/blog.

Body Outlaws: Rewriting the Rules of Beauty and Body Image edited by Ophira Edut, foreword by Rebecca Walker. $15.95, 1-58005-108-1. Filled with honesty and humor, this groundbreaking anthology offers stories by women who have chosen to ignore, subvert, or redefine the dominate beauty standard in order to feel at home in their bodies.

About Face: 25 Women Write about What They See When They Look in the Mirror edited by Anne Burt and Christina Baker Kline. $15.95, 1-58005-246-0. 25 women writers candidly examine their own faces—and each face has a story to tell.

30 Second Seduction: How Advertisers Lure Women Through Flattery, Flirtation, and Manipulation by Andrea Gardner. $ 14.95, 1-58005-212-6. *Marketplace* reporter Andrea Gardner focuses on the many ways that advertising targets women and how those ads affect decisions, purchases, and everyday life.

The Bigger, The Better, The Tighter the Sweater edited by Samantha Schoech and Lisa Taggart. $14.95, 1-58005-210-X. A refreshingly honest and funny collection of essays on how women view their bodies.

The Nonrunner's Marathon Guide for Women: Get Off Your Butt and On with Your Training by Dawn Dais. $14.95, 1-58005-205-3. Cheer on your inner runner with this accessible, funny, and practical guide.

Better Than I Ever Expected: Straight Talk About Sex after Sixty by Joan Price. $15.95, 1-58005-152-9. A warm, witty, and honest book that contends with the challenges and celebrates the delights of older-life sexuality.